Digital Imaging

A Primer for Radiographers, Radiologists and Health Care Professionals

D1288640

Digital Imaging

A Primer for Radiographers, Radiologists and Health Care Professionals

Edited By

Jason Oakley

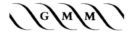

Contents

List of Contributors in Alphabetical Order

Dr Martin Benwell
Department of Radiography
Institute of Health Sciences
City University London

Marco Crispini
IT Consultant

Dr Michael Farquharson
Department of Radiography
Institute of Health Sciences
City University London

Terry Jones BSc
PACS Administrator
Portsmouth NHS Hospitals Trust
Portsmouth

Jason Oakley MSc
Department of Radiography
Institute of Health Sciences
City University London

Acknowledgements

This book would not have been possible without the contributions of many individuals and thanks are due all of them who have been listed here in no particular order.

Thank you to Mr Roger Hicks and the Staff at the Department of Radiography, City University for their support and especially to Delia Hayes, Dr Martin Benwell and Dr Mic Farquharson.

Thank you to the staff at the Department of Radiography, Queen Alexandra Hospital, Portsmouth for their invaluable help, support and encouragement over the years.

Thank you to the staff of the Medical Physics Department, Portsmouth NHS Hospitals Trust for their advice and guidance.

Thank you to the authors for finding the time amongst their busy schedules to contribute.

Thank you to FUJI for enabling the use of images within this book.

This book is dedicated to my wife Michaela and my daughters Molly and Mia for giving me the support to see it through to its completion.

Any questions or comments on the topic of digital imaging will be gladly received and in the first instance should be sent for the attention of the editor, Jason Oakley at gavins@greenwich-medical.co.uk with the subject 'book question'. A reply will follow as soon as commitments allow.

GENERAL INTRODUCTION
Jason Oakley

This book has been written to fulfil a need that has become apparent in the modern National Health Service (NHS). With the constant advancement and availability of technology, the drive towards the electronic patient record (EPR) and the electronic health record (EHR) for General Practitioners (GPs) the need for modern medical professionals to be conversant with information technology has never been so great. From the combined experiences of the authors it was apparent that no single book sought to bring together the core of information that was required to achieve this and also to act as a reference for the future.

When considering the target audience the content was primarily aimed at radiographers and radiologists either involved in the procurement process for new equipment, undertaking a course in digital imaging or frustrated at their general lack of knowledge with regards to the technology that they were already using. However any health care professional with an interest in the field of digital medical imaging will find this book a valuable resource. This would include doctors and nurses utilising Picture Archiving and Communications Systems (PACS) either within clinics or on wards and also health care professionals remote from the secondary care facilities of a hospital, such as General Practitioners (GPs).

The aim of this book is not to turn its reader into a computer engineer and there are many fine books that together with further study can achieve this end. It is more of a one-stop shop for the concise and pertinent information that experience has shown as necessary.

As PACS become more wide spread the impact of imaging technology will affect a much wider and diverse population of staff, and with this will come new challenges in education and training, many of which can be addressed by the subject matter herein.

In a field as diverse as medical imaging and as complex as computing this modest book cannot hope to address in depth all that might be required for a person to be termed an 'expert', but it will lay at the fingertips of the reader the key facts.

It has been written to fulfil three roles;

Firstly to be a book that could be read cover-to-cover to provide a thorough grounding in digital medical imaging. Secondly as a reference book to be referred to for key facts, and the highlighted boxes at the beginning of some of the sections, along with the glossary, aim to achieve this.

Finally it is hoped that the reader will find this book compatible with the philosophy of continuing professional development (CPD). The final chapter of this book is divided into multiple choice question (MCQ) sections followed by a list of answers. These sections test the knowledge of the reader on the main facts from many of the sections of the book. Radiographers, Radiologists and others will all benefit from this section.

Each section will be followed by a list of references and sources used in the chapter's construction. Any web references will also carry a brief description of the sites contents and a summary of its most useful elements. As with all web based references the longevity of them cannot be guaranteed.

The first chapter will explore the history of the development of computers along side the evolution of radiography and radiology. This chapter has been included to demonstrate the very rapid rate of change that both radiology and computing have undertaken in the last twenty years.

The second chapter will look at some basic concepts that the reader will have to have a grasp of before reading the subsequent sections of the book. The material includes descriptions of binary, hexadecimal and magnetic domains amongst others.

Chapter three explores the basic equipment that may be encountered. The field of equipment is, however, huge and this means that every manufacturers piece of equipment may differ slightly in design, function or use.

Chapter four explores the standards (interface standards such as DICOM and HL7) used in healthcare imaging and information systems to allow interface between different systems. Again this chapter will barely touch the surface of what is a complex area. However, the reader will at least have an understanding of what the standards do, if not exactly how it is achieved.

Chapters five, six and seven look at how the information generated within a department is managed, looking at the Radiology Information System (RIS), the PACS and the entire network of communications within a digital hospital. This interfacing of systems together is probably one of the most important and useful aspects of modern medical imaging.

Chapter eight explores how medical images may be processed to enhance their diagnostic usefulness. The very topical issue of the potential uses of compression for medical images is also discussed here. Chapter nine follows on from this with an in depth look at what makes up image quality and how it can be measured.

Chapter ten follows on from the image processing and quality and looks at common parameters that are used to automatically alter the appearance of images.

The practical experiences of both radiographers and radiologists are explored in chapter eleven, giving those about to install systems the benefits of others experiences. Discussion is frank and the disadvantages as well as the potential advantages included.

A number of the important documents and websites are discussed in chapter twelve, including the potential impact of the human rights act. This chapter is not meant to replace the original documents, but rather to give the reader an idea of where to find certain information amidst the forest that is information technology.

Finally the future of digital imaging in radiology will be discussed, but this chapter will no doubt be almost out of date by the time the reader reads it due to the rapid advances being made.

An extensive glossary drawn from the chapters is included at the end as a source of ready reference.

This book will not look at all digital imaging acquisition devices, such as Computed Tomography (CT), Magnetic Resonance Imaging (MRI), Ultrasound (US) or Nuclear Medicine (NM). These imaging devices are complex in their own right and deserve the more thorough coverage a dedicated book provides.

There is no doubt that these are exciting times to be working in health care, and the changes that are possible through the management and exchange of digital data are many fold. In the modern National Health Service (NHS) not a single role will be unaffected by the installation and implementation of these new and emerging technologies, but with the aid of this book the change will at least be an informed one.

1: A BRIEF HISTORY OF RADIOGRAPHY AND COMPUTERS

Jason Oakley

When you consider the relatively brief history of radiography and radiology the technological advances that have been made in medical imaging are nothing short of astounding. The range of diagnostic imaging tools that the modern physician has at their disposal is vast, and more often than not taken for granted.

Yet despite advances in its own right there is little doubt that with out the parallel advances in computing technology medical imaging would not have advanced as far as it has. As the history of computers shows they too would not have been developed if it were not for the industrial and political pressures that have prevailed throughout history.

Computer technology has also now reached a stage where it has been able to make use of existing infrastructures (such as the copper wire telephone network) to continually extend it uses and to reach more individuals. This has resulted in the acceptance of computers by many areas of society and this has in turn driven the technology forwards. In example the worldwide embracing of the Internet has led to the need for faster and more reliable connections that in turn has led to the current move towards broadband connection, even for domestic use.

FROM SIMPLE BEGINNINGS

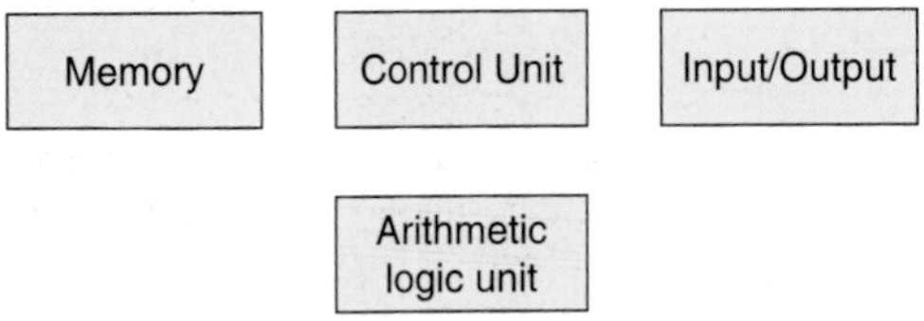

Figure 1 – Simple schematic of a computer

Computers have primarily four components and these can be seen right back to the earliest times in the form of the abacus. The abacus originated from Mesopotamia in about 3500BC, but it still fulfils all of the above functions, albeit in a combined fashion.

The control unit, the part of the computer that controls how the information is handled is the physically structured formation of the beads, and the human mind. The arithmetic logic unit is the rows of beads arranged into a known format and the knowledge of how to use them. The input device is the moving of the beads by the user from data acquired and the output device is the final display of beads.

Memory is also the final display of the beads, but this is of course volatile (the earliest type of random access memory (RAM) that could be lost by shaking or tipping the abacus) and more permanent methods of storing data such as writing were employed to save data.

The abacus remained the primary method of calculating for many years, despite many historical figures speculating on the possibility of storing information or calculating figures using a mechanical device. In 1642 Blaise Pascal (1623–1662) invented a simple adding and subtraction machine but at the time such inventions were considered as interesting, but not essential.

As the world became far more economically and financially driven there was a demand for reliable automated calculating machines but it was not until Gottfried Leibniz (1646–1716) began to theorise that this might be made easier using binary code (using only two numbers, 0 and 1) that developments were made. Leibniz worked upon the principle of keeping calculations as simple as possible, or using a finger to represent on or off, and it is from this that the term *digit*al is now derived.

The 18th Century and the industrial revolution led to mass production on a previously unseen scale. With it came the pressure for an ever-increasing output to drive the profits even higher. Basile Bouchon first created a loom that relied upon punched cards to control the pattern around 1725. The famed Jacquard Loom invented by Joseph-Marie Jacquard (1754–1834) perfected this technique in 1801. This was the development of the first program to control a device, but was not a computer because no calculations actually took place.

Charles Babbage (1791–1871) developed the first true equivalent to a modern computer known as the analytical engine (difference engine) in 1835. The machine used gears and cogs to carry out the calculations, but the machine was itself controlled by a card with holes punched in it. Despite its potential the cost spiralled out of control and the full machine was never finished. However, the wheels had been set in motion for the computer era.

In the late 1830s the telegraph began to allow long distance communication utilising a single wire along which signals could be sent using a code developed by Samuel Morse (1791–1872). This technology rapidly spread with the laying of the first submarine cross channel cable in 1851 and the first transatlantic cable in the early 1860s.

This was rapidly followed by the teleprinter, a device that printed a readable tape from the incoming signal, and in 1876 Alexander Graham Bell (1847–1922) gave the first public demonstration of the telephone, opening up a new era in communications. During the same period the typewriter in the form that we now know it became popular, with the QWERTY keyboard being developed to keep commonly used letters apart to prevent the keys jamming during rapid typing.

Herman Hollerith (1860–1929) developed a tabulating machine to allow the processing of data from the 1890 US census. His machine took the concept of punched cards utilised by the weaving industry to control a calculating machine, effectively introducing the idea of using computers to process large amounts of information. The success of this led to the creation of the Tabulating and Recording Company, which in 1924 combined with others to form IBM (International Business Machines).

John Logie Baird (1888–1946) developed the first mechanical method of scanning an image and as such has been remembered as the creator of television (circa 1926), but it was Vladimir Zworykin who produced the first television camera in 1929 that utilised an electron beam to scan the image and produce a waveform that could be sent to a modified cathode ray tube that then displayed the image.

It was during the 1930s that the Americans and the Germans began to independently develop the idea of the electro-mechanical computer. Alan Turing (1912–54) published a paper in 1936 defining what would become known as a 'Universal Computer'. This was a device that could be programmed to carry out any function that the user desired.

Konrad Zuse is attributed with developing the first computer with a stored program, the Z3, which was developed for military purposes but did not survive World War II. The idea of the stored program had originally been conceived by John Von Neumann (1903–57). In 1943 the Colossus machine was built to break German messages sent in code form and utilised 1500 vacuum tubes to process the information via a program that was created using patch cables that could be moved to alter the sequence.

At the same time in the United States (US) the Harvard Mark 1 was created in conjunction with Howard Aiken. The Mark 1 measured $15.3 \times 2.4 \times 0.6$m. These machines utilised thermionic valves, which were far quicker than mechanical switches, but by today's standards were still very limited in what they could achieve despite their size.

The first true electronic computer was developed in 1948 at Manchester University and in 1949 the Ferranti 1 became the first computer to be specifically developed for the commercial market. In the US Von Neumman's ideas were developed by John Mauchly (1907–80) and J Presper Eckert (1919–1995) who developed the first fully automated electronic computer called ENIAC and released the first commercially available computer UNIVAC in 1951. This machine was also the first to replace punched cards with magnetic tape.

The development of the transistor, which is a solid-state semiconductor, in the late 1940s reduced the cost and increased the speed of computers. It also improved their reliability and by 1953 the first transistor computer had been developed, again by Manchester University. The late 1950s saw the development of the world's first 'super computer' and the first international computer language, FORTRAN.

In 1958 the first Integrated Circuit (IC) was manufactured. This is now known as a microchip, normally made of silicon, which via a complex process is built to contain all of the electronics required for a computer. They can be created to process or to store information.

1963 saw the release of the 7 bit ASCII (American standard code for information interchange). This was the first real standard that would allow all computers to exchange textual information. Each potential value from 0–127 was allocated a value on the keyboard. The international version, ISO-7 was implemented in 1973, but it is the US version that is still used in most computers to define the basic character set.

In 1968 Intel released the first 1 kilobyte memory chip. This was the year before the first men went to the moon. One of the prime considerations of the Apollo design team was how to keep the weight of any computer down, and this resulted in an erasable memory on board of only a few kilobytes.

In 1972 Intel released the 4004, the first microprocessor. This directly led to the development of the microcomputer and started the development of the cheap and reliable computers that are in use today,

From the late 1960s a phenomena known as Moore's Law is said to be in place. In about 1965 one of the founders of the Intel Corporation commented on the fact that the amount of memory that could be fitted into a unit area had doubled nearly every year. This is now true for a period of about eighteen months, and in the same period the price of the memory roughly halves, meaning that newer systems come out at the same price as the systems available eighteen months previously.

If we consider the history of radiography to this point the developments have been far less revolutionary. Indeed from the discovery of x-rays by Wilhelm Roentgen in 1895 very little has changed in the fundamentals of what is done. A stream of electrons are still drawn by a large potential difference towards a target of a high atomic number where interactions take place that produce a large amount of heat and a small amount (<5%) of x-rays. This stream of x-rays effectively casts a shadow of whatever is placed in its way and this shadow can be recorded on a suitable medium.

Fluoroscopy was first developed in 1896 by Thomas Eddison (1847–1931) (amongst others) and in the same year Michael Pupin (1858–1935) combined Clacium-Tungstate screens with photographic film to dramatically reduce the time of exposure required to produce an image, although glass plates were used for some time.

In 1913 William Coolidge (1873–1975) made the x-ray tube more efficient by making the inside of the tubes a true vacuum. In 1918 exposures were further reduced with the introduction of duplitised film and intensifying screen combinations. The dangers of x-rays were only now being taken seriously and the 1920s saw the development of a philosophy of 'Radiation Health' in the United States.

In 1933 blue tint was first added to the base layer of films by Du-Pont to enhance their subjective appearance, and over the next two decades most of the developments were to do with film construction and quality. The first image intensifier and television system was released in 1955, reducing the dose previously received from looking directly into phosphor screens. 1956 saw the introduction of the first automatic processing system by Kodak. The rare earth screens released by 3M in 1973 made a large impact on doses and these types of screens are still in use.

It was in the 1970s that the worlds of computers and medical imaging first began to meet. Computers had made the whole concept of imaging a slice within a volume possible due to the vast number of simultaneous equations required for back projection (in excess of 25,000). In 1974 EMI released the first computed tomography (CT) scanner for clinical use, developed by Sir Godfrey Hounsfield. This was the start of the digital era within medical imaging.

With the development of magnetic resonance imaging (MRI) in the late 1970s and its introduction into clinical use in the 1980s a whole new field of medical imaging was being developed that brought with it the need for image storage and manipulation. Only the increasing specifications of computers has enabled the volume helical CT and volume MRI imaging selling so many systems to become a reality.

In the early eighties the National Electrical Manufacturers Association (NEMA) in association with the American College of Radiographers developed the first NEMA standard and in 1985 the initial standard was released. Its aim was to ensure that all images produced in medical imaging were at least transferable between systems, if only at a basic level. This was the standard that would go on to become the DICOM (Digital Imaging and Communications in Medicine) standard that is in use today (see Chapter 4 – Interface Standards)

In 1978 the first analogue wave form medical image was converted to a digital image allowing a whole new era of digital radiography to become possible, including digital subtraction angiography (DSA). Fuji, utilising phosphor storage plates and a laser imager to print the images, introduced phosphor plate technology in 1983 and true digital imaging utilising charged coupled devices (CCDs) was introduced by many companies during the 1990s

The equipment in use today in a modern digital imaging department is a real fusion between the independent histories of computers and radiography. One could not exist without the other, and they are prime examples of how one technology can take what has been developed in another and utilise it to further its own ends.

REFERENCES

BOOKS

Byrd W 1995 **Understanding Computers** Jain Publishing Company

Watteville A de, Naughton S 1998 **Advanced Information Technology** Heinemann

Wilson B 1996 **Information Technology: The Basics** Macmillan

WWW

http://www.hq.nasa.gov/office/pao/History/computers/Ch2-5.html
   Interesting online book at the NASA site on the history of computers in spaceflight.

http://www.ccspr.com/samples/rad-time.htm
   A timeline of the history of x-rays from Kodak

http://www.cnde.iastate.edu/ncce/RT_CC/Sec.1.1/Sec.1.1.html
   A history of radiography

http://www.isbe.man.ac.uk/personal/dellard/dje/history_mri/history%20of%20mri.htm
   A brief history of MRI

http://www.imaginis.com/faq/milestones.asp
   History of diagnosis and diagnostics

http://medical.nema.org/
   Official DICOM website

http://www.ee.ryerson.ca:8080/~elf/abacus/
   The Abacus and the art of calculating with beads

http://www.sciencemuseum.org.uk/picturelibrary/index.asp
   A useful resource of science based images

http://www.maxmon.com/history.htm
   A review of the history of computers

http://ei.cs.vt.edu/~history/
   Resource on the history of computers

http://www.digitalcentury.com/encyclo/update/comp_hd.html
   Jones Telecommunications and Multimedia Encyclopaedia

http://www.cbi.umn.edu/
   The Charles Babbage Institute – a good resource for information on the history of hardware and software

http://www.computerhistory.org/
   Excellent from the Computer Museum History Centre

2: THE BASICS

Jason Oakley

INTRODUCTION

This chapter will revisit some of the basic theory that it is important to have a grasp of in order to understand the way in which the equipment and technology works. This chapter will assume little prior knowledge and as such may well be revision to a number of professional groups. More information on the specific subjects can be found utilising the book and web references included at the end of the section

Much of the information included may be familiar in a superficial way but by the end of this section the reader will have a much fuller understanding of many of the terms used in digital imaging

BINARY CODE

Society currently works in decimal. That means that we count numbers using ten individual digits to make up all numbers. Any number can be made up of combinations of these ten numbers (0–9). See table 1 for examples

The decimal system most probably developed because humans have ten digits with which to count (eight fingers and two thumbs) and it was therefore the most natural number base for us to work with. This is known as Base 10, but it is perfectly possible, and in many cases easier or more efficient to work with other bases, such as Base 2.

Base 10 would be very complex for a computer to replicate (and therefore prohibitively expensive), and would also require extensive electronics to allow a computer to store one of a possible ten states (0–9). It is very much easier for an electronic device such as a computer to register something as being on or off, 1 or 0, and this is why the binary system is used. An electronic switch can be used to represent these two states and by linking them together many different variables can be stored.

In exactly the same way as the decimal system is capable of creating any number so is the binary system, but by only using two digits (hence the name **bi**nary). See table 2 for examples of how this works in practice. Because we are working in binary the columns are represented by the 2^x ($2^1, 2^2, 2^3$ etc) in the same way that the columns in decimal are represented by 10^x ($10^1, 10^2, 10^3$ etc).

This may seem longer and unnecessarily complex to us but for a computer this is the simplest and most reliable from in which data can be handled, stored and transmitted.

It is the fact that the columns are formed by the formula 2^x that results in the strange figures that we associate with image resolution and storage in medical imaging. For example a computed tomography (CT) image is 512×512 pixels (262144 or 2^{18}) and has a bit depth of 8 ($2^8 = 256$ grey scale image).

These individual parts are called bits of data, and eight bits are normally referred to as a byte. These slightly odd figures lead to an anomaly when looking at larger figures (i.e. a Megabyte is not actually a 1,000,000 bytes, but is in fact 1 048 576 bytes). Table 3 sums up the relationship of these figures for storage.

In table 3 you will note that the symbol for kilo is k (lower case) to agree with SI Unit recommendations, however it may be seen written as K. The large B is used to identify bytes, and the small b to identify bits. If you connect to the Internet and hover your mouse icon over the modem connection icon it will tell you how

Table 1 – decimal examples

Original	Hundreds	Tens	Units	Resultant
9	0	0	9	9
101	1	0	1	101
937	9	3	7	937

Table 2 – binary examples

Original	512	256	128	64	32	16	8	4	2	Units	Resultant
9	0	0	0	0	0	0	1	0	0	1	0000001001
101	0	0	0	1	1	0	0	1	0	1	0001100101
937	1	1	1	0	1	0	1	0	0	1	1110101001

Table 3 – comparison of binary and decimal

Bytes	Power	Derived Unit	Symbol
1 bit		1b	
4 bits		1 nibble	
8 bits		1 byte	1B
1024	2^{10}	1 kilobyte	1kB
1 048 576	2^{20}	1 megabyte	1MB
1 073 741 824	2^{30}	1 gigabyte	1GB
1 099 511 627 776	2^{40}	1 terabyte	1TB
1 125 899 906 842 624	2^{50}	1 petabyte	1PB

many kbs are being received and sent. This is kilobits per second, not bytes.

The smallest unit in binary language is the bit, derived from *BI*nary digi*T*. The next larger unit is made up of four bits and known as a nibble, although this is not commonly used. More commonly eight bits are used and this is known as a byte. Having eight bits to a byte seems to have no firm origin other than experimental choice. Each byte is therefore made of eight bits that can be in the state 1 or 0. This gives us 2^8 or 256 combinations ranging from 0 to 255. To represent the decimal number 256 would require a 9 bit system. Let us use the decimal number 234 and convert this to decimal (many scientific calculators, including the Microsoft calculator in Windows can convert to binary).

11101010

The bit is often described as having a least significant bit (lsb) and a most significant bit (msb). The four bits to the right are described as the least significant nibble (lsn), and are made up of the four lowest value units. Conversely the bit to the far left is described as the most significant bit (msb), and is part of the most significant nibble (msn).

So what can these bits and bytes be used to record? They were originally used to record textual information. The ASCII (American standard code for information interchange) was mentioned briefly in the history of computers. It allocates the combination of a seven bit system to the characters on the keyboard, e.g.

65 A
66 B
67 C
68 D

Different numbers were needed to record the upper and lower case letters, numbers themselves and certain characters that are commonly used in textual information. The ASCII code (and adaptations of it) is the most common code that computers now use to store information to either the hard disk or the removable storage media (e.g. CD-R)

On a modern system each character will be represented on an 8-bit system (because 8 bits is the now the most common component of modern computers – the byte). If you have a Windows based system open up your notepad program in accessories and type the word 'four'. This will be made up of four bytes of data. Save this file to the desk top of your computer, close notepad and then right click on the icon and from the pop up window that appears select properties. One of the bits of information that will be displayed is the file size and this will be 4-bytes. The file size if the file is saved to a disk will be much larger as there will be other information that has to be sent with the simple textual data to allow the file to be opened that will often dwarf the actual textual information.

As previously mentioned it is the fact that the columns in our binary system are formed by the formula 2^x that results in the strange figures that we associate with image resolution in medical imaging. In our previous example of a computed tomography (CT) image the matrix size was 512 × 512 pixels (262144 or 2^{18}) and the bit depth 8 ($2^8 = 256$ grey level image).

In this example the total storage requirement for this image (without compression) is 512 × 512bytes (each byte already has eight bits available to store the necessary number of grey scales), so 512 × 512 = 262144. If we divide this figure by 1024 we can determine the number of kB required for the image. 262144/1024 = 256kB.

You can test this effect in a similar way to looking at textual information. Using any image manipulation program (such as Adobe Photoshop or CorelDraw) open up any image and resample it at 512 × 512 pixels. Change the image to an 8bit depth grey scale image and then save it as a bitmap (*.BMP) to the desktop of the computer. Close the program and then right click on the image icon and from the pop up menu select properties. The image will be just in excess of 256kB. Again the file size once saved to a disk will be much larger due to other information required by the computer to read the file.

The bit depth required depends upon the number of grey levels or the number of colours that need to be stored. Conventional film is the equivalent of a 10 bit system, and thus is capable of representing 1024 grey levels. Table 4 summarises the number of variables available for a variety of bit depths.

Table 4 – Bit depth compared to variables

Bit Depth	Power	No of variables
8	2^8	256
9	2^{19}	512
10	2^{10}	1024
11	2^{11}	2048
12	2^{12}	4096
13	2^{13}	8192
14	2^{14}	16384
15	2^{15}	32768
20	2^{20}	1048576
30	2^{30}	1073741824
40	2^{40}	1099511627776

HEXADECIMAL

The only problem with binary is that to represent very large numbers binary requires a very large number of columns. This large number of columns results in very long strings of binary digits. To avoid this a system known as Hexadecimal is used to represent long numbers and thus reduce the amount of data that needs to be stored.

Hexadecimal is a Base 16 system. Binary is Base 2 and we normally function in the real world in the Base of 10. The 16 digits are represented by the number 0–9 and the letters A–F, giving 16 variables in each column. This gives rise to the seemingly strange codes that appear on computer screens in the form 00F4:1E00

(The colon separates the code up into readable sections).

Table 5 demonstrates the differing length of digits required for decimal, binary and hexadecimal.

The MS Windows based system comes with a calculator (under accessories) that can convert any number to both binary and hexadecimal. Next time you come across one of these numbers input them into the calculator and see what the actual number was, and how long it would have been if it not been in hexadecimal.

THE DIGITAL IMAGE

So what is a digital Image?

The signal coming into a television set is continuous, varying in intensity over a period of time (fig 1.)

These varying peaks and troughs correspond to differing intensities on the final image. This waveform is used to vary the intensity of the electron beam in the cathode ray tube and thus vary the brightness of the phosphor at the point that it strikes (see Chapter 3, Equipment – Monitors for more detail.)

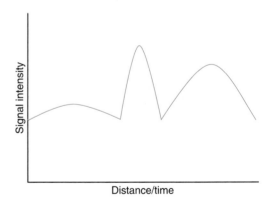

Figure 1 – An analogue waveform

Table 5 – Binary, decimal and hexadecimal compared

Name	Base	Number	Length
Binary	Base 2	1000000000000000000000000000000	31
Decimal	Base 10	1073741824	10
Hexadecimal	Base 16	4000:0000	8

This waveform is known as an analogue signal, and because it is a waveform it is prone to interference or loss of information during transmission. This results in a decreased signal to noise ratio (SNR) and a degradation of image quality. In the case of a television set this can be seen if a traditional aerial is not aligned accurately.

A digital image can be thought of as different because every pixel is made up of a discrete value, and not from a continuous wave form. A digital image is a string of binary numbers (0s and 1s) and this fact makes transmission very much less likely to experience problems, and if there is a problem in transmission the receiving software should be able to establish that an error in transmission has occurred.

A digital signal can be produced in a number of ways. Firstly the image may be acquired as an analogue waveform. This waveform may then be sampled at discrete and constant units of time. This is known as sampling the signal and can be done using an analogue to digital converter. The rate of sampling determines the resolution of the final image. If we take the same waveform as shown in figure 1 and sample it using large discrete units we obtain a digital representation (figure 2). However the sampling rate is so large that the original image seems very different.

If we increase the sampling rate we get a much more accurate representation of the original waveform. The more often we sample the waveform the higher the image resolution, and the larger the file size in terms of bits. See figure 3.

The other factor that sampling affects, and perhaps the most important, is image quality. Figure 4 shows the affects of sampling an image

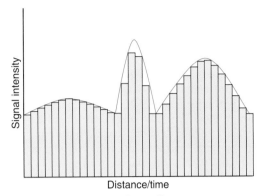

Figure 3 – Higher rate of sampling

to fit a matrix 512×512 (A), 128×128(B) and 32×32(C).

The level of sampling must be adequate for the purposes for which the final digital image is intended. For example, if the image you are acquiring is going to be used for a thumbnail image on a web site, and will only be shown at 32×32 pixels then acquiring at anymore than this will result in the image taking up more memory than is required for its purpose. Figure 5 shows the 32×32 image at 100%.

Note that the borders appear much smoother than they would if the image was magnified. Whilst the image is crude it is a very small file size and would be of use in circumstances where image size and not image quality was of prime importance.

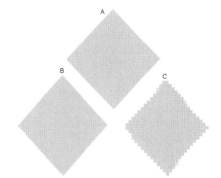

Figure 4 – Various sampling rates of an image

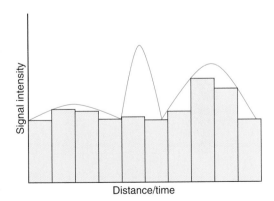

Figure 2 – Under sampling of waveform

Figure 5 – 32×32 matrix image at 100%

NYQUIST THEOREM

Nyquist theorem states that any system should sample at double the highest frequency that is present within an object if that object is to be represented at the appropriate frequency. Figure 6 shows the effect of sampling at the same frequency as the object, which is half the required frequency under Nyquist theorem.

If the sampling rate is doubled then the actual frequency within the image is recorded far more accurately (figure 7).

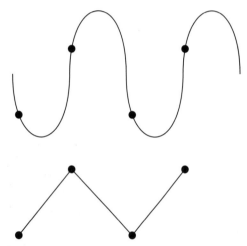

Figure 6 – Effect of sampling at lower than the Nyquist Frequency

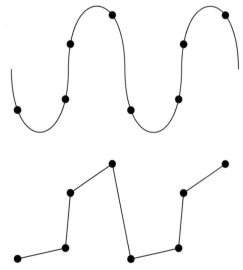

Figure 7 – The effect of sampling at double the highest frequency within the data (Nyquist Frequency)

If this is not done then the frequency will be represented at a frequency lower than it really is (known as aliasing). Conversely if the signal is over sampled then the file size will be unnecessarily large. Nyquist theorem and its implications will be further discussed under Chapter 9 – Image Quality.

The alternative to sampling an analogue waveform and digitising it is to directly acquire the data in digital format. This is by far the most expensive technology at the moment (discussed under Chapter 3 – Equipment). A useful analogy is the difference between taking a photograph (an analogue image) and then scanning it into a computer, and using a digital camera to acquire a picture directly. Both these processes fulfil the same function but one does it more conveniently and with less steps that may introduce errors and that may also cause image degradation to take place. Methods of acquisition utilising both direct an indirect technologies are dealt with in the equipment section.

An image made of discrete units has to have several attributes associated with it to allow us to view and manipulate it. As previously discussed most medical images tend to be acquired in a matrix that is to the power of 2 i.e. $2^{18} = 512 \times 512$ matrix, utilised in CT. As an example of the properties of an image we will look at a 2^{12} image matrix (64×64) with an eight bit depth ($2^8 = 256$ grey scale). See figure 8.

The image is made up of 4096 pixels arranged in 64 rows of 64 pixels. Each pixel has a position which is a determined by x and y – (x,y). Each pixel can also be allocated one of 256 grey scales or a function. This means that each pixel of an image can be represented by $f(x,y)$.

Whilst at the moment the majority of medical

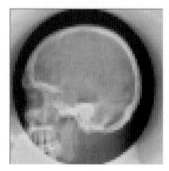

Figure 8 – 64×64 lateral skull

images utilise only grey scales to display data there is a move towards incorporating more false colour into images to enhance detail. Many reconstructions in CT & MRI now utilise colour to define different structures and colour Doppler incorporates colour onto a grey scale image. To store colour information a single value is not enough. Information needs to be stored for the red, green and blue component that makes up the final pixel of the image.

If each pixel has 2^8 bits associated with each of the colours (256 blue, 256 green, 256 red) that would give $256 \times 256 \times 256 = 65536$ different colours that could be displayed. However this will have an effect on the size of the image that is being stored. In the example of a 256x256 matrix 8 bit depth grey scale image the file will be 512kB. A colour image will be three times this size.

CT and MRI images have another important feature inherent in them, and that is that each pixel also has depth. When either sequential or volume data are acquired the subsequent reconstruction of the image results in an averaging of the data in that volume to produce what has now to be termed a voxel (a pixel that has volume).

This averaging has been long known as the partial volume affect in CT and is best explained using this modality although it applies equally to any volume acquisition technique. Figure 10 shows a 10mm reconstruction of a single CT pixel. The slice has gone through 50% bone and 50% soft tissue with CT numbers of 1000 and 20 respectively. The resultant value (f) of the pixel will be an average of these values, in this case 510, which is not accurate in either case.

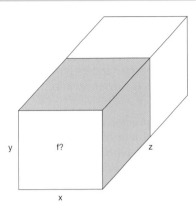

Figure 10 – Partial volume effect

Reducing the width of the slice reconstructed or acquired can lessen partial volume effects. However, this has the effect of reducing the signal to noise ratio (SNR) within the pixel which will reduce the quality of the image. As with all medical imaging it is careful use of all parameters that gives optimum image quality

Data acquired in series or volumes also has to have spatial information recorded, usually in the form of table position. This allows the images to be viewed in the correct order and also for manipulations to be carried out on multiple images in order to produce multi-planar reconstructions (MPRs), maximum intensity projections (MIPS) and other 3D rendering techniques.

One further value that may also be recorded is that of temporal (time) position. This is required when acquiring a series of images over a period of time when it is the time that is important and not the position (images may be at one or at multiple locations). This would be important in modalities such as nuclear medicine, ultrasound and angiography.

Utilising pixels or voxels with their associated digital values allows us to do many things to the image, including manipulations, accurate storage, accurate retrieval and image transfer between systems.

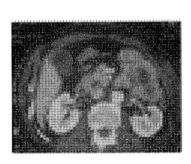
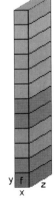

Figure 9 – CT data showing voxels

THE IMAGE FILE

An image file is comprised of two distinct elements, the file header and then the data set. The header contains the essential information of the file.

- Patient information associated with image – this is a vital part of the image. If this information is not reliably transferred then the image cannot be subsequently linked to that patient.
- Total file size – this allows the receiving computer to ensure that all of the information was received.
- Start and end points of data file – this allows the computer to know when the file is starting and where the file ends.
- Matrix size – if the matrix size is included then the x,y co-ordinates of the pixels within the image do not need to be sent. The computer can take the grey level values and fill the matrix in a known fashion so that the end result is the full image.
- Grey level or colour (RGB) – allows the computer to display the images appropriately.

The chapter on Interface Standards (4) will expand more on the many fields that are now required for a medical image to contain within its header.

Following the header is the data file that contains the information about the spatial location (if required) and associated levels.

MANIPULATIONS

Various mathematical functions can be carried out on these numbers allowing the appearance of the image to be altered to reveal or enhance information (Chapter 8 – Image Processing). These may result in a simple change of brightness to complex image manipulation using preset look up tables (LUTs).

STORAGE

A stored analogue signal is subject to the same potential degradation in image quality as a transmitted analogue image. A stored digital image, by storing only 0s and 1s should be of exactly the same quality as the original image (unless manipulations were carried out prior to storage). This results in a more efficient method for the long-term storage of data.

Error checking can be built into software to ensure that information is always accurately recalled and multiple backup copies can be made to prevent accidental loss from a single location.

MAGNETIC DOMAIN THEORY

Whilst there is a move towards optical systems (which will be discussed fully under the Chapter 3 – Equipment) the hard drive and floppy disk drive (3.5 inch) are still very evident. There is also a resurgence in the use of magnetic tape and knowledge of basic magnetic domain theory is essential. Magneto-optical systems are also commonplace that utilise both lasers and magnetic fields to accurately and more permanently write information to a disc.

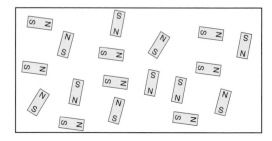

Figure 11 – Randomly orientated domains

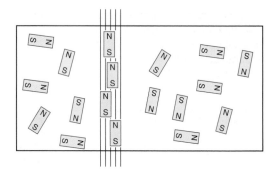

Figure 12 – Aligned magnetic domains in a magnetic field

Magnetic domain theory states that within a solid magnetic substance there are many microscopic areas that act like little magnets. These are normally randomly orientated and thus exhibit no magnetic properties (figure 11).

If the tiny domains are exposed to a magnetic field they will align with the magnetic field (figure 12).

When the magnetic field is removed the tiny domains will maintain this orientation and the information is thus permanently stored. This is in essence how information is stored onto all magnetic media. To read the data the tape is read by a device that can sense the change of magnetic field within the tape. This is then converted into the signal that the computer can use.

Analogue media, such as audiotape, record a continuous waveform. Digital media record a series of 1 and 0s. Hard drives are very precisely made and sealed environments in order that the magnetic domains that can be written and read are as small as possible and maximum data can be stored. Tapes are capable of storing less information because the magnetic domains have to be larger.

To erase a tape a randomly varying magnetic field can be used to 'scramble' any data that was stored there thus making it illegible to any system.

BANDWIDTH

This a very current topic with the media excitedly reporting on the current reduction of costs in 'broadband' Internet connection and the potential for a 'Broadband Britain'. An understanding of bandwidth is important to understand some of the factors that will be referred to in subsequent chapters.

Bandwidth has two distinct definitions;

ANALOGUE BANDWIDTH

An analogue signal is a waveform. A wave has a specific wavelength, with high frequencies having a shorter wavelength and lower frequencies having a longer wavelength. The range of frequencies (from low to high) that an analogue system can deal with determines its analogue bandwidth. The larger the range of frequencies that are possible on the system, the broader the bandwidth.

DIGITAL BANDWIDTH

Bandwidth is also used to describe the transfer of digital information. In this case it would be quoted as bits per second (bps) or bytes per second (Bps). The speed of any transfer or receiving system will be governed by the component with the lowest bandwidth.

Most UK Internet users are still connected to POTS (plain old telephone system) but there is now a growing move towards other dedicated Internet connections. This is the case with broadband that utilises a broader digital bandwidth to speed up the Internet connection.

ISDN lines (Integrated Services Digital Network) utilise two POTS to send information at double the fastest modem rates without having to use a dedicated Internet connection. Other systems also utilise an unequal transfer and receive rate. This is done because most users of the Internet receive vast amounts of information (viewing pages, downloading documents), but send very little by comparison. Asymmetric Digital Subscriber Line (ADSL) allows a faster downstream rate (on to your hard drive) than upstream rate (from your computer). This permits maximum performance of the system in normal use.

DIGITAL IMAGING AND DOSE

When computed radiography was first used clinically, the doses were very slightly higher than those from comparable film screen systems and this extra dose was justified by the increased diagnostic potential of the image via manipulation and reduction in repeats due to over exposure.

Doses soon became equal and more modern systems do allow a minimal dose saving. However this saving should not be exploited without a thorough examination of the subsequent image quality and this will be discussed more fully in the Chapter 9 – Image Quality.

A potential danger with digital imaging systems is the use of consistently higher exposures than are necessary to ensure an image of diagnostic quality every time. The imaging system will automatically manipulate the image to display what appears to be a perfectly exposed radiograph that would have in fact been over penetrated on a conventional film/screen system. It is very important that whatever system is installed that the doses are closely monitored to ensure that all of the benefits of digital imaging are reaped.

HUMAN COMPUTER INTERACTIONS

The capabilities of human beings to adapt to new environments and work patterns is enormous, but the introduction of computer systems should be seen as a very radical step that might require a large change in mind set for many individuals.

Of the utmost importance when changing from conventional systems to digital systems is the need for initial and then continuing training in the new technology. A method of assessing staff is also important to ensure that they are coping with the technology as well as they appear to be. Never assume that all members of staff will be able to use all of the equipment

Other issues that will have to be considered are those of health and safety and these will be discussed under Chapter 12 entitled 'Summary of Important Documents'. There are many computer users around the country who are now unable to work as a result of work related upper limb disorders (incorrectly previously called repetitive strain injury [RSI]). All risk assessment should be carried out on an individual basis and not at a departmental level.

It is strongly recommended that if other parts of the book seem unfamiliar to the reader that time is taken out to research these areas prior to continuing. This will enable the reader to gain the most from the time spent with this book.

REFERENCES AND SOURCES

BOOKS

Boden L 1995 **Mastering CD ROM technology** John Wiley and Sons

Byrd W 1995 **Understanding Computers** Jain Publishing Company

Robertson I 1995 **Hard Drives Made Simple** Butterworth Heinemann Ltd

Watteville A de, Naughton S 1998 **Advanced Information Technology** Heinemann

Wilson B 1996 **Information Technology: The Basics** Macmillan

WWW

http://www.howstuffworks.com
  Very useful site with information on almost everything that you can imagine

http://www.gcn.ou.edu/~jahern/comp_aps/bits_bytes.html
  Excellent tutorials on the basics of bits and bytes

www.newcastle.edu.au/department/av/bilby/number_sys.htm
  Information on different number systems

http://www.webopedia.com
  Very extensive web based encyclopaedia

http://www.diagnosticimaging.com/digitalradiography/role-lowers.shtml
  Information on CR vs DR

http://www.gemedicalsystems.com/rad/xr/education/
  General Electric educational site for radiography

3: EQUIPMENT

Jason Oakley

INTRODUCTION

Whilst an engineers knowledge of the equipment is not necessary to operate equipment it is useful for those involved with modern medical imaging equipment to be aware of the technologies that go to make up the digital solution to imaging in the modern National Health Service (NHS). It is the combined authors' experience that some individuals within any area will become interested and over time extremely knowledgeable on the individual systems and this chapter will give those people a good grounding.

This chapter will only look at the most common pieces of equipment and technologies that will be encountered and where possible relate them to the actual working environment, addressing issues that will need to be considered during procurement. Rather than covering each piece of equipment in depth it will identify the pertinent points to aid the reader identify areas of further study.

As previously mentioned this book will not cover the acquisition technology behind computed tomography (CT), magnetic resonance imaging (MRI), nuclear medicine (NM) or ultrasound (US). These modalities are complex in their own right and deserve the attention that can only be afforded to them in a single dedicated book. This chapter will be dedicated to equipment that is not found in conventional radiology and radiography text books.

However each of the modalities that have not been covered will produce an image that is digital in nature and much of this chapter (such as monitor technology and hardcopy devices) will still be relevant. Other chapters are relevant to all modalities.

Because of the length of this chapter and the amount of information within it there will be three multiple-choice question sections dedicated to it in the MCQ section of the book. This will allow the reader a more thorough assimilation of the data contained.

The first piece of equipment that will be looked at will be the workstation and the peripheral devices that attach to it. Visual display equipment (monitors etc.) will be discussed later.

WORKSTATION COMPONENTS

INTRODUCTION

Modern computer systems tend to no longer be of the proprietary version. Proprietary was the term used to describe equipment produced by a single manufacturer that relied upon their own software and often their own storage devices. Files were stored in the manufacturers own format and many of these devices are now unreadable.

In recent years there has been a move to software programmes that run on a standard or high specification personal computers (PC). Two main types of PC exist, those based on the IBM format and those on the Apple Macintosh. This section will look at the main components of any IBM PC workstation that might be part of a networked system. Other components that may not be found in the hospital setting will also be included for completeness as future uses for these devices may become apparent. Under the final chapter, Future Developments, the latest equipment will be described, along with its potential uses in the clinical environment.

Workstations come in many forms, varying in the quality of the monitor, speed of processor

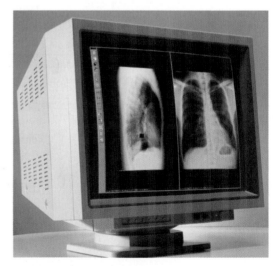

Figure 1 – Fuji Work Station
(picture courtesy of Fuji)

and the type of input/output devices that are used. The cost will vary greatly depending again on the quality of the monitor etc, and a recurrent theme in modern medical imaging is that the equipment should be fit for the purpose for which it is intended to be used. This theme should be borne in mind throughout this section.

The architecture of a system refers to the general set-up of the system. A computer with a common architecture will be useful for allowing components to be readily exchanged and for expansions and upgrades to be as simple as possible.

Open architecture normally refers to a Picture Archiving and Communications Systems (PACS) set-up where each of the components can easily be replaced by a similar device albeit from a different manufacturer. A closed architecture system would require an identical piece of equipment to replace the piece that is being removed.

WORKSTATION SET-UP

The following schematic diagram shows the main components of any PC based workstation.

Each of the areas will be considered in turn, identifying the important points within each area.

Power Supply

Whilst most computers now run from conventional mains supply there are specific issues

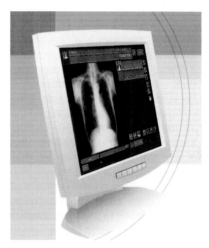

Figure 3 – Fuji QA workstation
(image courtesy of FUJI)

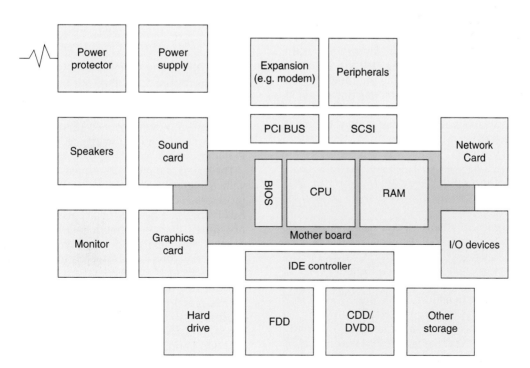

Figure 2 – Schematic diagram of a PC

within medical imaging that need to be considered. For example if the power supply to a computer were to be lost for even a moment the volatile memory (random access memory – RAM) would instantly be lost. If this happened in the home whilst writing a letter all that would be lost would be time but in Radiology the potential exists for an image to be lost and the patient to subsequently have to be re x-rayed.

The solution to this problem is a power protector, also known as a UPS (un-interruptible power supply). These are devices with large batteries that detect when a power interruption is occurring and ensure the smooth transition to the battery supply without the loss of data. Whilst the power supply within them is limited (10–15 minutes) this is long enough for a controlled shut down of the equipment to be commenced, thus protecting the data stored there. A UPS will also protect the equipment from power surges that may be caused by large pieces of equipment being turned off or by faults in the local supply.

The cost of a UPS is determined by the length of time that they will protect the system for. The longer they protect for, the heavier they will also be, as a larger battery will be present. A UPS gives the users time to perform a controlled shut down of the systems, avoiding the loss of data, but this does assume that there is a user around to initiate the shut down at the prompt of the UPS. Intelligent UPS systems perform the same function but will initiate the shutdown of the system whilst the battery still has power, avoiding problems that may result from the users not being aware that the power supply has been interrupted.

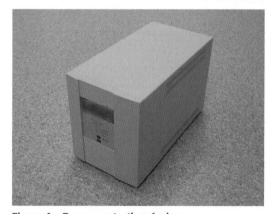

Figure 4 – Power protection device

Mother Board

This is the name given to the main circuit board in the computer (hence its name) through which all of the main components are either a part of or are connected to. It also allows further expansion of the volatile memory (RAM) and replacement of individual components without replacing the entire system.

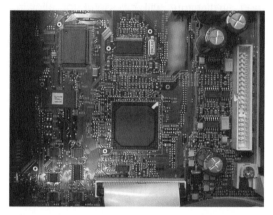

Figure 5 – Mother board with components in situ

The motherboard holds the following components:

CPU

Central Processing Unit – in the same way that our brain oversees all that our bodies do, the CPU does the same. It is responsible for controlling everything that the computer does. This is now more commonly termed simply the (micro) processor and comes in many forms such as the Pentium.

The speed of a processor is measured in Hertz, with a higher cycle being faster for a specific processor. For example an old 486 processor (still being used by NASA due to its reliability) is not faster than a Pentium II 236 processor, despite the Pentium's apparent processing speed being lower. The speed is determined by the system clock, which contains a quartz crystal to precisely control the timing of electrical impulses and therefore the speed at which the processor can process information

The processor utilises the system memory (RAM) to perform logic and arithmetic functions, and as such the microprocessor and the RAM are inextricably linked, with each having a part

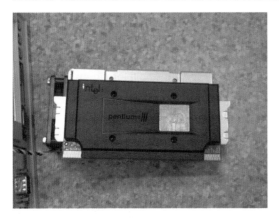

Figure 6 – Processor in situ

to play in the overall systems performance. If the processor is slow or if there is only limited access to memory then the computer system will be slow.

Processors are now easily upgraded, allowing the speed of the computer to be improved without replacing the whole computer. In the same way RAM expansion cards can easily be slotted into the motherboard allowing the amount of RAM available to be increased to again speed up the processing abilities of the computer system.

Arithmetic Logic Unit

The Arithmetic Logic Unit (ALU) is actually part of the processor and is responsible for carrying out mathematical functions such as adding and subtracting. It also responsible for what are known as logical functions, such as searching for numbers larger than a known variable.

For complex applications that require complex mathematical computations a maths co-processor can be added that will contribute to the work of the ALU and again improve the speed at which large calculations can be made.

System Memory

The system memory, also known as the primary memory of the computer, is more commonly known as RAM (Random Access Memory) and will be referred to as RAM throughout this book. RAM is a very fast type of temporary storage for data that the processor is directly connected to. It is made up of either transistors or capacitors, which are simple electronic devices. They can be in one of two states, either on or off to represent

a 1 or a 0 in binary code. With modern technology the number of these that can be squeezed onto one chip is very large.

RAM can be further classified as dynamic (needing constant refreshing), or static (where the charge is constant). Whilst static is faster it can hold less memory and is disproportionately expensive, so most systems at this time utilise dynamic RAM.

The RAM is divided up into specific areas where the computer stores the data that it is currently being used. It is known as volatile memory because if the power supply is interrupted the information stored in the transistors or capacitors is immediately lost. There is one important part of the RAM known as the CMOS (complimentary metal-oxide semiconductor) that is constant because it is connected to a small battery. This portion of the RAM is used to remember how the computer system is set up and the location of the drives and peripherals. If this portion of the RAM fails then the computer will fail to start properly.

All computer systems will require some of the RAM to be taken up by the operating program, such as MS-DOS (Microsoft Data Operating System). If the DOS utilises a graphical user interface (GUI) then the amount of memory taken up will be much larger. As an example if the system in use has 64Mb of RAM then at least 8MB will be taken up by the GUI DOS. A further 8MB may be taken up by software applications to display incoming images. This leaves approximately 48MB of free RAM to display images.

A single chest x-ray might be in the region of 8–32MB, so for the display and manipulation of images large amounts of RAM are needed. If not enough RAM is available then the CPU will designate a part of the hard drive of the computer as *virtual memory*. This will act as more RAM (sometimes called virtual RAM) but the hard drive is much slower than the RAM and thus the computer's performance will suffer.

To improve the speed of a computer it is often more effective to increase the RAM than to change the processor.

BIOS

Basic Input/Output System – this is a basic read only memory (ROM) that contains the instructions that allow the computer to turn itself on and communicate with the other pieces of equipment such as the keyboard. Also referred to as ROM BIOS.

Without the BIOS the computer would never be able to enter boot up mode. When a computer is turned on it first utilises the BIOS to check the system before searching the A:/ drive for a boot up program. If one is not found the other drives are then searched. When a boot up program is found the control of the system is then handed over from the BIOS to the software (the DOS).

The term 'boot up' is derived from the phrase 'to pull yourself up by your boot straps' and refers to the computer starting itself up.

Other pieces of dedicated equipment may also have their own ROM BIOS, such as graphics cards, which may be utilised in digital radiography systems to accelerate the display of complex graphics.

Internal Bus

A bus is a link between two components of a system that allows them to exchange signals. These are normally arranged in parallel for faster data transfer i.e. rather than each bit of information being sent separately they can be sent at the same time, or in parallel. This is a term that is also used when talking about network connections.

PCI BUS

PCI stands for Peripheral Component Interconnect. This is usually a series of slots in the motherboard to allow devices to be attached quickly and easily. Internal modems, memory expansions and other devices can be added in this way without having to alter the construction of the computer. The type of motherboard in situ will determine the number of devices that can be added via this route.

Secondary Storage

Secondary storage refers to all other types of memory that a computer might use (not RAM). Secondary memory can be further divided into those that are physically fixed within the computer such as the hard drive and types of removable storage such as floppy disks and CD-ROMs.

This memory is permanent in that it is not lost if the power is interrupted and in many cases can be written and read again and again. The most common types of storage media will be explained under *Storage*.

Controller Cards

Controller cards are multipurpose devices that control the operation of hard drives, disk drives and some parallel port devices. Some drives will have controller cards built into them and will not rely on a central control device.

Buffer

A buffer is a section of the RAM that is sectioned off to provide a temporary storage area for data that has been held up. For example a modern processor is capable of processing information faster than it can be written to the floppy disk drive. The processor will write information to the buffer that will then send the data to the floppy disk drive when it is free to receive it. The processor is then freed up to carry out other tasks whilst the buffer takes over the job of writing the data to the disk.

Some equipment comes with built in memory that acts as a buffer outside of the computer, again to allow the computer to be freed up to carry out other tasks. Such accessory memory increases the cost of any equipment.

Sound Card

A soundcard is a device that allows the conversion of digital sound into an analogue waveform to allow the sound to be heard via a set of speakers. The soundcard also allows incoming analogue signals to be converted into digital form to permit their storage and manipulation on a computer system.

Medical uses of this may seem limited at the moment but as picture archiving and communications systems (PACS) expands to embrace the philosophy of the Electronic Patient Record (EPR) then sound will become another record to be kept on a patient. An example might be Doppler studies, cardiac sounds etc.

There is also a move towards dictated reporting direct onto a computer system, which then converts the spoken word automatically into text. The next step on from this is to have the computer store the spoken word as well and for the viewer of the image be able to hear the radiologist discussing the image as well as reading the written report.

Graphics Card

The graphics card or visual graphics adapter does the same for the monitor as the sound card does for the speakers. A graphics card takes the digital information stored on the computer and converts it into a form that the display device can use. This may be a true digital monitor or a conventional cathode ray tube that will utilise an analogue waveform to generate the image (this chapter – **VISUAL DISPLAY EQUIPMENT**).

It is important that the graphics card is matched to the monitor or certain signals may not be properly transmitted resulting in incorrect or incomplete image display. Graphics cards utilise Video RAM in the same way that the processors utilise the system RAM. With large image files it is very important that large quantities of Video RAM are available to speed up the processing and subsequent display of the image. Graphics cards are necessary in modern systems to allow them to run at full resolution and at maximum colour.

3D graphics cards, which are most commonly associated with the games industry, will soon have applications within medical imaging for the display of volume rendering techniques currently being used primarily in computed tomography (CT) and magnetic resonance imaging (MRI).

Network Card

Network cards are also known as network interface cards. For the computer to be connected to the network the appropriate network card must be in place to allow it to see and talk to the rest of the network. It is the network card that is responsible for receiving and sending data to the network in a format that the network can handle and that can then be received by other systems on the network.

Modem

Most hospital systems will not utilise a modem for communication with other systems, including access to the Internet. However when the data is being sent to a remote source, such as a radiologist at home the link may be via a modem. The main problem with modems is that they are limited in the amount of data that can be sent per unit time. This means that large image files may take far too long to be sent for an opinion to be given in real time on a set of images. The modem is therefore included here only for completeness.

The word modem is short for *mo*dulator and *dem*odulator. A modem is a device that can utilise a POTS (plain old telephone system) to gain access to a remote computer. The modem then converts a digital data stream into an analogue waveform that can be transmitted over the POTS or other system. This conversion of digital data to analogue signal is known as modulation.

The modem at the receiving end then takes the analogue waveform and converts it back into a digital data stream that the computer can utilise. This conversion from an analogue signal to digital data is known as demodulation.

Modems operate at a variety of speeds and may be integral or peripheral. Integral means that the component (modem or otherwise) is within the main case of the computer. A peripheral device is a stand-alone device that is connected to the computer via a cable attached to a port on the computer.

I/O devices

It is of course essential that the user is able to interface with the computer in some way. There are currently a number of devices that allow the user to do this. These devices connect via the many ports on the back of the computer and these will be looked at first before listing the many input/output devices that connect to them. Figure 7 shows an example of the many ports that can be seen on the back of a computer.

Ports

A port is a connection point for input/output devices that allows direct communications with the corresponding circuitry on the motherboard. They are usually capable of being either input or output and will normally be of specific shapes to ensure that the appropriate piece of equipment is plugged into the right port.

The ports will also have either a male or female type connection. Male connections are made of pins that are arranged in a particular fashion. A female port is comprised of holes that will receive the pins on the connection device

Serial Ports

A serial port is a connection to the motherboard that will allow only relatively slow transfer of data in a sequential fashion. They are sometimes termed sequential ports or connections.

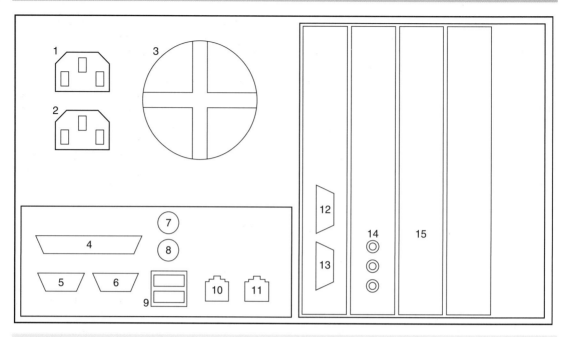

Key

1	Power input	9	USB Port
2	Power output for connection to monitor	10	Network Connection
3	Cooling Fan	11	Second Network Connection
4	Parellel Port	12	Monitor Connection
5	Serial Port	13	Second Monitor Connection
6	Serial Port	14	Sound Card with inputs for Microphone and MIDI and output for Speakers
7	Keyboard Connection	15	Spare expansion slot cover
8	Mouse Connection		

Figure 7 – Connections for input/output devices

Only one bit of information can be sent at a time.

Parallel Ports

A parallel port is a connection that will allow a separate channel for each of the bits of data to allow them to be sent in parallel, or simultaneously. This speeds up the rate at which data can be transferred between devices.

USB

Universal Serial Bus. This is a very simple connection device that allows very rapid transfer of data between the main computer system and a peripheral device. Any device that is connected to the computer via the USB should be 'hot swappable' meaning that multiple devices maybe interchanged without turning the computer off and restarting it with the new device attached.

USB connections seem likely to replace both serial and parallel connections over the next few years.

SCSI

Small Computer System Interface (SCSI) is the hardware component that allows up to seven peripheral devices, such as scanners to communicate with and be controlled by the computer.

Keyboard

A keyboard is far more complex than it looks, containing a large wire matrix whose connections are formed when the keys on the keyboard are depressed. Inside a keyboard is a small microprocessor that senses which key or combination of keys has been pressed. This is then turned into a code (often the ASCII code) that is then sent to the computer to indicate the character that should be displayed or the action that the computer should carry out. A memory buffer within the keyboard controls the rate at which information is sent.

Within the processor the information is linked to specific characters depending on the type of keyboard specified in the software. Keyboards are not generally 'hot' swappable, that is they cannot be swapped whilst the computer is still on. Installation of a new keyboard needs to take place when the computer is off.

The keyboard is the device that allows the user to input text-based information and comes in many different forms, although common types are the ZT and PS/2. They may have additional keys, such as function keys or be more compact for specific uses.

Most keyboards are based on the QWERTY layout that was originally designed for the first manual typewriters whose mechanics made them prone to jamming unless commonly used letters were kept apart. Other keyboard layouts exist that are theoretically more efficient, but lack the familiarity of the QWERTY layout.

Mouse

The mouse, like a keyboard is most commonly an electro-mechanical device, but whereas the keyboard allows the input of characters the mouse allows manipulation of the screen environment. This can mean moving a cursor to click on a 'button' or picking up and dragging large or small images.

The mouse is known as a 'pointing device' and is now the most commonly used of these. Other pointing devices that are still available, but not as common, include laser pens, joysticks (popular in the games industry) and data tablets (popular in computer aided design–CAD).

The electro-mechanical version of the mouse involves a ball that when rolled turns wheels that correspond to the x and y direction of the cursor on the screen. These tiny wheels turn larger wheels with perforations in their perimeter that interrupt the light being sent by an infrared light emitting diode (LED) to an infrared light sensitive diode. This information is trans-

ferred via the mouse's own processor to the computer where the operating system translates the information into the movement of the cursor on the screen.

The pressing of the keys (there may be up to 8) again registers in the mouse's processor and a signal is sent to the operating system and the function is carried out that corresponds to this signal. A mouse may come with a variety of buttons to allow different actions to be performed and the software being used normally determines the function of these buttons.

The mouse is normally connected to the computer by a cable, although infrared models (tailless) are available. The latest models have no moving parts but sense the movement via sensors, thus prolonging the life of the mouse. These are completely electronic devices.

The mouse is not normally a 'hot swappable' component and if disconnected whilst the computer is on and then reattached the system must be rebooted to sense that the mouse is again connected.

A *trackerball* is essentially the same as a mouse except that the device itself remains static and a ball moved within it by the operator.

Barcode readers

Barcodes are very much a part of everyday life, being the primary means of identifying many consumer products. This proliferation of the technology means that barcodes are tried and tested technology for the exchange of data between two systems that cannot connect directly. The barcode has come to have many uses in what are often termed the hotel services within hospitals, such as catering, laundry and security provisions. However they also have uses within the imaging department.

For example if there is a problem with the interface between the radiology information system (RIS) and the computed radiography (CR) or digital radiography (DR) system one solution is to enable your RIS to print barcodes (a relatively simple program that converts the ASCII code into a barcode that other systems can read) to enable faster and more accurate inputting of patient data. This removes the problems associated with multiple inputting of patient data, such as typing errors, and also removes the need for expensive and sometimes unworkable interfaces between older systems. It is this type of interface problem that DICOM and HL7 (two standards that are discussed in Chapter 4 – Interface Standards) set out to avoid.

Computers find it very hard to read text, as anyone who has attempted optical character recognition (OCR) will attest to. Instead barcodes can be produced that computers can read quickly using reading devices.

A barcode is made up of black lines of varying widths and white spaces of varying widths, each which represents a number. When the reading device scans the barcode a signal is produced that will correspond to the black and white spaces on the barcode. The computer can then either convert the signal directly into the information required or into a code that can be converted to get the correct information. A confirmatory bleep confirms that reading has taken place

There are several type of barcode reader that all achieve the same end result. The wand utilises a bright light that is reflected back or absorbed by the barcode and detected by a charge-coupled device (CCD) within the reader. The signal to and from the reader is analogue and this signal is converted using a standalone processor (the wand is normally connected to a small box that then connects to the computer or to the network) into a signal that the operating system in the computer can use.

A barcode 'gun' utilises a bank of CCDs to read the barcode as a strip of light is flashed across them. The multiple readings from the CCDs are used to create the waveform instead of the movement of the wand. Essentially they perform the same task, although the barcode wand relies far more on user technique than the gun.

Laser scanners also exist and these allow barcodes to be scanned at a distance (10–20cm) rather than having to be close to the reader. This again improves user compliance but also means that the techniques used to scan the barcode must be more accurate. Whilst barcode readers are designed to make the inputting of data more accurate they do not prevent the user scanning the wrong barcode and thus inputting incorrect data. There is still no substitute for checking that patient data is correct on every patient in the same way as was done when imaging with conventional film/screen systems.

SOFTWARE

Software is the essential ingredient that tells the computer to do the things that we want it to. Without the software the computer would be little more than a collection of metal, plastics and ceramics. There are many types of software packages available and this section will look briefly at only the generic types and not individual programs.

Health Informatics (HI) and the use of computers by all members of staff is a reality within the National Health Service and as such there are already moves to ensure key competencies such as ability to word process a document or send e-mail. These skills are being incorporated into a qualification known as the European Computer Driving Licence (ECDL) that may well become part of every member of staffs initial training.

Operating System (OS)

Once the computer has booted itself up from the BIOS and performed the power on self test (POST) the overall control of the computer is then handed over to the operating system (OS). This is a program that is able to handle all of the hardware in a consistent fashion which means that the other software programs being run on the computer can concentrate on doing what they were designed to do, such as manipulate an image. These other programs then rely upon the operating system to print the image once the application has requested that it does so.

The operating system is also responsible for the multi-tasking element of the computer. When several applications are running the OS designates a certain amount of time to each of the programs that are waiting for processes to be carried out on the CPU. It also ensures that adequate time has been given for that part of the task to be carried out to prevent time being wasted on calculation or functions that are never completed

Examples of operating systems are Windows, UNIX and Apple Mac, although there are many others available. Text based systems (such as DOS) are faster but they do not have the user interoperability that is associated with the graphical user interfaces (GUIs) such as Microsoft Windows. However the use of GUIs to control the DOS does mean that the systems operate slower.

Applications

An application program has a specific role to perform, such as to acquire and manipulate images. It will depend upon the operating system for certain functions such as storing data and printing hard copies. Windows is a graphical user interface (GUI) for a data operating system. Word for windows is an application, which again uses a graphical user interface to run the various functions that the program is capable of.

As previously mentioned the GUI makes a system slower because the instruction given in the windows environment has to then be translated into the actual command in the DOS environment. However the consistency of the GUI means that many users find it easier to move between applications because of the familiarity with the general layout. Common functions are also easy to find.

Viruses

Viruses are sequences of code that have been deliberately designed to do a certain amount of damage to the data stored within a personal computer (PC) system. The virus might simply copy itself onto your hard drive or it might replicate itself and e-mail copies of itself to all those in your e-mail address book where its offspring will repeat the process. More malicious viruses can completely obliterate all the data stored on your computer by reformatting all of the drives.

Viruses require the user to do something to execute the file such as open e-mail or execute a file that then triggers the virus. This can happen without any warning from the computer so the user may be unaware of a problem.

Worms are similar to viruses but do not need user intervention to propagate and can be far more destructive and since the introduction of broadband seem to be proliferating.

With stand alone digital imaging systems the chance of a virus infecting the system was slight, but with fully integrated systems the danger becomes very large, especially when individual machines are being used to search the Internet, download e-mails and access image archives.

An effective policy for dealing with the potential threat of a virus is essential, and this may involve the use of a software protection package or the use of a firewall to prevent certain types of files being downloaded to the system. Files that are commonly infected include word documents and executable e-mail attachments.

Computers are very complex and the last section is designed to give the reader a working knowledge of the basics. The next section will look at storage. Storage may be integral within the workstation, known as local storage, or part of a separate system.

STORAGE MEDIA

INTRODUCTION

With the digital age comes the inescapable problem of how to store the large amounts of data that are going to be generated every day. The numbers of variables that can affect the choice of storage media are long and this section will endeavour to fulfil two objectives;

1. **Identify the criteria for choosing a storage media.**

2. **Identify the main types of storage available.**

CRITERIA FOR CHOOSING STORAGE MEDIA

This section has been put together using several references and also the combined experiences of the authors with regards to storage issues.

1. Temporary or Permanent Storage?

It is important to know what the main function of the storage media is going to be. Is it going to be to store a single months work permanently online to enable rapid access or is it going to immediately archive to the long-term storage? If fast access were required for the last month then a Redundant Array of Independent Disks (RAID) would be ideal for this purpose. If the system were going to store images straight to long-term storage then an optical disk (CD, DVD or 5.5 inch OD) would be ideal as retrieval is relatively fast and juke box systems exist to allow multiple disks to be online within a few moments. If the storage media is required to only back up data files, and quick retrieval is not essential then a digital tape might be the ideal choice due to its cost and durability.

2. Image File Size

This may seem obvious but is vitally important that consideration is made to the number of images that a medium can hold. If many larger files are required to be stored (such as is the case in a PACS environment) then the number of images per disk is important. It may be even more important if your remit is to have five years of work online within five minutes. This can be achieved using any number of retrieval devices (carousel or jukebox etc.) but if the capacity of your chosen storage medium is only twenty images per disk and your workload will fill two disks per day, then five years of work online would require 3650 discs.

Compression may be the answer, but this has problems that need to be addressed prior to its use (see Image Processing- Compression).

3. Image Retrieval

How is it intended for offline images to be retrieved? This could be as basic as a person taking a phone call, finding the appropriate disc or tape and then cueing the media up to be viewed online. This has many problems, such as backlog of work, errors in storage or misfiling, availability of staff, and the issue of providing an out of hours service.

A better solution might be an automated retrieval device, but this will limit your choice of storage media and will have cost and maintenance implications. However it removes many of the problems associated with human input, and deals with the out of hour's provision.

In general, storage media can be defined as sequential or direct access. A tape is sequential and several minutes may be required for the tape to be spooled to the correct position to allow the data required to be retrieved. An optical disc can jump to the correct part of the disc to retrieve the data instantaneously but the images are likely to cost slightly more to store on this medium.

4. Storage times

How long does the choice of media take to write the data to the storage media? Will this affect the imaging systems capability to show new images that are being received? Some systems will allow the user the option to store only at quiet periods, such as at night, thus reducing the potential impact of large data writing during the day. This option comes with the associated risk of losing data that has not been backed up if there is a major failure prior to writing to the storage media.

5. Read Times

This is a variable that can be addressed by the technology that you are willing to pay for. The speed of a system is invariably related to its cost, and a happy medium must be found between the length of time the end users are willing to wait for an image to be recalled and the cost of the system.

The read times are further complicated by the speed of the network system. No matter how fast you make the reading device and the computer that is going to use the information, if the network is inadequate or too busy the apparent retrieval time will seem very long.

A sensible compromise is that the retrieval time is likely to be short for images that have been recently taken, but longer for images that were taken some time ago. These two different scenarios can be addressed through the use of a large temporary storage system for 'current' images (the RAID) and a slower retrieval system for offline images. The number of image that can be considered 'current' will depend upon the size of the RAID that is considered economically reasonable. This will vary from a few days to a few months

6. Longevity

How long are the images to be kept for? There is little doubt that digitally stored images will out live the current requirements for conventional film storage (5–10 years) but what is the potential for the storage of images? Certainly, a CD could be expected to last for fifty years if stored carefully. This has implications under the Data Protection Act (See Chapter 12 – Summary of Important Documents) which states that data should not be kept for any longer than absolutely necessary, and it may be possible to have disks that have information on them that is necessary and other data that could be deleted if it was possible to delete it.

Another issue under longevity is the long-term readability of the storage medium (future proofing).

7. Durability

If the wear and tear on the storage media is going to be minimal then this will not be an issue, but if the last five years of disks are going to be constantly exchanged using a jukebox system then a certain amount of durability must be expected. The reading device must also reflect this where a better quality system will be able to read a poorer quality disk more easily, and be less likely to damage the disks due to failure.

8. Location

The location of the storage media is of prime importance. If the stored data and the imaging system are in the same place and are destroyed by fire all of the data is lost. Current trends are to store data in specially constructed rooms that are designed to deal will all but the most devastating of disasters.

There are also exists the possibility of double backing up all data to a remote secure location.

9. Future proofing

An issue prior to DICOM was that if the images were stored using proprietary software, and the imaging device later changed, the images could no longer be read. DICOM has gone some way to solving this problem, but technology may result in certain media being discarded. There are many unusual systems on the market, some of which are very popular at the moment, but not as popular as the CD-ROM.

The 1980s saw the demise of Betamax video, despite its superior image quality. The secret is to select a storage media that is popular and has a well-established standard that allows multiple vendors to produce and use it. A good example of this is the 3.25-inch floppy disk that has been around for many years. VHS triumphed over Betamax for the same reasons.

10. Cost

Cost effectiveness does not mean choosing the cheapest alternative (or it should not). The accurate definition of cost effectiveness is choosing the most appropriate medium after considering all of the above requirements. Storage is an area where the wrong choice will have long-term effects on an imaging department's capabilities. There are several points that will be mentioned

several times throughout the course of this book and one of those is that PACS can only expect to be received well if it is implemented properly and with appropriate funding. Users do not want worse or even the same from a new system. They want better.

TYPES OF STORAGE MEDIA

Storage media can broadly be divided into three areas,
- Magneto systems
- Optical systems
- Magneto-optical systems

Magneto Systems

Magnet domain theory was explored under Chapter Two – The Basics. Magnetic systems are a cheap and reliable form of memory storage and will remain a familiar part of computing for some time to come. This section will explore the most common types of media. It will not cover videotapes because whilst they are a magnetic recording medium they do not record digital data. In modern imaging systems a digital cine series does not require a videotape to record it but instead is stored as a stream of digital signals. Videotape and traditional audiotape are both analogue recording mediums.

Floppy Disk Drives

IN BRIEF

FDD	Floppy Disk Drive
HD	High Density
Capacity	1.44MB (2MB unformatted)
Speed	Depends upon drive write speed
Size	87.5mm D × 4mm
Cost	< £0.20 approx
Cost per 1MB	£0.14 approx
Advantages	Good for easy data transfer, but not images
Disadvantages	Very small memory size and prone to corruption

Introduction

Floppy disks have been included for complete-ness but they are of little use in the radiology environment other than for the quick and easy transfer of word processed documents or spread sheets. They do however explain the basic concepts of all storage, those being:

1) The formatting of the area, on which data is to be stored,
2) The creation of a directory so that a computer reading the data knows where to find the data and
3) The storage of the actual data itself.

Construction

Floppy disk drives are made of a very thin sheet of plastic coated on *both* sides in a magnetic material. The actual storage area is circular and this is held in a rigid plastic case for protection, with a sliding cover at one end that prevents foreign material gathering on the magnetic surface and subsequently transferring to the read head of the disk drive.

The material used to coat the plastic is very similar to that used for tape storage, but has the advantage of the drive being able to jump to data that has been stored rather than having to fast forward to that point in the tape. This is known as *Direct Access Storage.*

Data Storage

The storage surface of the disk is formatted by the computer into concentric rings, which are known as *tracks*. The disk is further divided into wedge shaped areas that segment the concentric rings into *sectors* (see figure 8)

Data is stored in these tracks and sectors, allowing the drive rapid access to all of the data. When the disk is formatted it is allocated a label that allows a computer reading the disk to ensure that the disk is present for all operations.

During formatting the disk is divided into four areas that will be used to store specific information. The File Allocation Table (FAT) contains a complete list of where all files are held on the disk and whilst the disk is in use a copy of this is kept in the system RAM for speed. The root directory is a map of where each file is stored utilising sub directories (a tree). A file can be

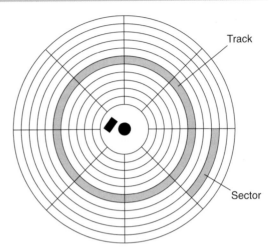

Figure 8 – Write area of a floppy disc

found by either method. Another of the allocated sections is the boot record and it is here that information is stored to allow a computer to boot up. The final area on the disk is the data storage area that is made up of the tracks and sectors.

Floppy Disk Drive

The floppy disk drive has a mechanical device that retracts the cover from the front of the cassette as it is inserted, revealing the disk beneath. Two heads are utilised to read/write both sides of the disk. The heads are not opposite each other, but are slightly offset to avoid the magnetic fields affecting with each other.

Data is written onto the disk as described in Chapter 2 – The Basics, magnetic domains. Floppy disks have the advantage of being able to be written and erased many times. They are also very cheap to manufacture, but their capacity is very small. A higher capacity disk known as a Zip Drive is available and relies upon the data being stored on a more expensive higher density disk. Zip drives are capable of storing hundreds of megabytes of data. However, because they still utilise magnetic domains to store the information they cannot achieve the density or fast read times of optical devices.

Hard Drives

IN BRIEF

HDD	Hard Disk Drive
Capacity	Typically 4–40GB
Speed	CPU delivery rate – 5–50MB/sec
Seek time	Time taken to find a file normally milliseconds
Size	Variable
Cost	£1.25 per GB
Cost per 1MB	< £0.01
Advantages	Relatively cheap, tried technology
Disadvantages	Non portable, and hardware more expensive than other mediums

Introduction

A hard disk is a computers main permanent memory storage area. It is known as a hard disk because the information stored is permanent (until deliberately deleted), not volatile like the RAM and is safe even when there is no power to the system. Hard drives are basically the same technology as floppy disks that can also be written to again and again

Construction

A hard disk is typically disc shaped and made of magnetic material impregnated into aluminium polished smooth in order to get maximum information on to its surface. It is also important that the read/write head is as close as possible to the surface for efficient transfer of data. The term 'crash' comes from the read/write head impacting the surface of the disk.

To increase the memory capacity several discs (known as platters) can be stored one on top of the other, each with its own read/write head. The head is attached to an arm that is capable of moving from the inside to the outside of the disk in 0.02s. The disk itself has a motor attached that rotates it in excess of 3500 rpm. This means that data can be found on the disk extremely quickly.

The hard drive is completely sealed to avoid any dirt, dust or debris getting inside and affecting the movement of the read/write head or damaging the surfaces of the platters.

Data Storage

Data storage is performed by altering the orientation of magnetic domains within the magnetic material. The amount of information stored on a hard disk can be enormous and will of course change regularly, so it cannot be stored in the linear fashion used for CD-ROMs or DVDs. Instead the disk is divided into Sectors and Tracks in the same way as a floppy disk.

A hard drive will also have a file allocation table and a root directory in the same way as a floppy disk will. The root directory is normally c:\ on a computer with one hard drive, and all of the files stored on it will stem from this. A practical example of this can be seen by using the explore facility of windows on any drive.

The drive will show a tree like structure of files stemming from the root directory. It is possible to create a partitioned drive where the computer will treat a single hard drive as a multiple drives.

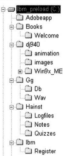

Figure 9 – Example of C:\ drive directory from Microsoft Windows 98

Magnetic Tape

IN BRIEF

DAT	Digital Audio Tape
DLT	Digital Linear Tape
Capacity	200+ MB
Speed	CPU delivery rate
Seek time	Variable depending upon where file is on tape
Size	Varies

Cost	5GB tape approx £20.00
Cost per 1MB	< £0.01
Advantages	Relatively cheap, tried technology. Large memory capacity – ideal for backup
Disadvantages	Indirect access, some concerns over robustness in frequent use. Also difficult to alter data

Introduction

Hard drives and floppy disks allow the read/write head to move directly to the area that needs to be read, meaning that data retrieval rates are very fast. However digital linear tape (DLT) is a reliable medium that is ideal for storing large amounts of data, and thus lends itself for the long the back up of data.

Tape units are also known as tape streamers or as cartridge units and can now be incorporated into jukebox systems that allow archives of multiple systems to be available rapidly.

Construction

Tape is made from a plastic tape coated with an iron oxide that is capable of being magnetised. The tape can vary in length and width depending on the exact type of tape being used.

Data Storage

Data is stored across the tape (see figure 10) by magnetising an area of magnetic tape, which is known as a 'spot'. A spot represents a 1 and an area with no magnetisation a 0. A complete character is written across the tape, so an 8bit system will have eight tracks plus an extra track that allows the computer to check that it has read the rest of the data correctly. A 10bit system will have eleven tracks. A complete character is known as a frame.

A complete set of data is known as a record

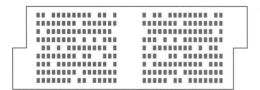

Figure 10 – Tape layout

and this will be followed by an inter-record gap (IRG) that signals the computer that that record has ended and another will begin. This gap also allows the tape reader a moment to slow down when it finds the end of the record prior to the one that it is searching for. Records that are related can be written together and this will improve the speed with which the data can be read.

Depending on the complexity of the tape reader it may have a single read/write head or a separate head for reading and another for writing data. Once data has been written it can be written over again but any alteration may not fit onto the gap left by the previous record and the new record will therefore normally be written at the end of the existing records. This results in patient data potentially occurring at several points in a single or multiple tapes that may again increase the retrieval time.

Tape does have the advantage of being able to hold large amounts of data but the sequential nature of its information means that data takes longer to retrieve than from a direct access device, such as a CD-ROM. Tape readers are now much faster with smaller IRGs and this has meant that the tape is reappearing as a viable alternative to more expensive technologies.

Optical Systems

The definition of an optical system is a system that uses light, normally in the form of a laser, to store and read the data.

CD-ROM, CD-R, CDRW & CD Drives

IN BRIEF

CD-ROM	Compact Disc Read Only Memory
CD-R	Compact Disc Recordable (WORM)
CD-RW	Compact Disc Re-Writable
Capacity	650–800MB
Speed	Depends upon drive write speed
Size	120mm D × 1.2mm
Cost	£0.20 approx
Cost per 1MB	< £0.01 approx
Advantages	Cheap, tried technology
Disadvantages	Only 20–100 images per disk (depending on compression), storage & retrieval issues

Introduction

Compact discs (CDs) are tried and tested technology that is now being used in the home to store personal data. CDs are a technology with which we are all familiar, but they do have some severe limitations if they are to be used to store uncompressed data. However they are now very inexpensive to manufacture.

All CD technology comes under the category of *optical storage media* by virtue of the fact that a laser is utilised to read (and in some cases write) the data. Magneto optical systems will be dealt with following CD and DVD technology.

CD Drives

There are two types of CD drive, the CD-ROM (compact disc read only memory) drive that only allows data to be read and the CD-R/RW that allows recording and rewriting. A laser is used in all three cases, but it is the temperature of the laser that is altered depending upon the exact recording medium.

To read the data the laser scans the track of information. The exact method of scanning depends upon the type of CD being used.

General Structure

A CD is a thin film of aluminium sandwiched between a piece of clear polycarbonate and a film of acetate in the shape of a disc 120mm x 1.2mm.

CD-ROM

The construction of a pre-made CD-ROM results in the data being already pressed into the polycarbonate layer in the form of bumps and troughs. The aluminium is then laid over this to reflect the laser to the optical pickup. This information is permanently stored and cannot be over written, destroyed or altered.

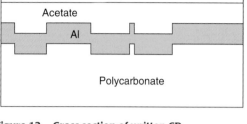

Figure 12 – Cross section of written CD

As the laser scans the track the bumps reflect the laser differently to the troughs, resulting in a varying signal with in the optical pick up. This varying signal corresponds to 0s and 1s in the stored data.

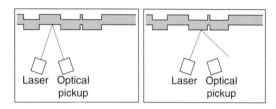

Figure 13 – Reading of data from CD-ROM

CD-R

The construction of CD-Rs differs because they have a layer of dye between the aluminium and the polycarbonate (which are made perfectly flat so they are no bumps or troughs. When data is written to the CD a higher power laser heats the area to be recorded and turns the dye black. This serves the same purpose as the bumps in the CD-ROM. Once the dye has been 'burnt' the information is permanently recorded.

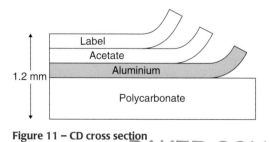

Figure 11 – CD cross section

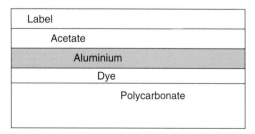

Figure 14 – Recordable CD structure

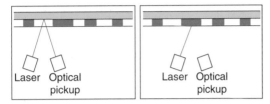

Figure 15 – CD-R data reading

CD-RW

The construction of CD-RWs differs by utilising a mixture of metals (antimony, indium, silver and tellurium) which when heated to different temperatures is either reflective or dull. In the same way as the CD-R the dull areas do not reflect the light. To re-write the crystals are reheated.

General Data Reading

The data on all CDs is written from the centre of the discs outwards in a single spiral track (very much like a record in reverse). This track is only 0.5 microns wide and nearly 5 km long.

However the diameter of the disc gets larger as the spiral moves out so the length of the track changes meaning that the data would be written and read at different speeds on the inner and outer edges of the CD if the disc were to rotate at the same speed.

To compensate for this effect a variable motor is employed which steps the revolutions down from 500 rpm in the centre to 350 rpm towards the outer edge. This allows the read or write rate to remain constant over the total area of the disc and ensure that maximum data can be stored.

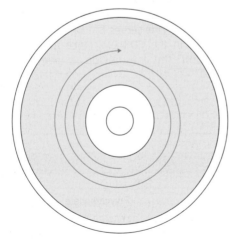

Figure 16 – CD track

The actual speed of data writing and reading depends upon the speed of the drive that you are using. All CDs have their read speed on the front as a simple multiple, 30× etc. This figure is derived from how many times faster the drive is than the first CD system that was made available by Philips and wrote at 150 kBs.

DVD

IN BRIEF

DVD	Digital Versatile Disk
Capacity	1GB+
Speed	Depends on drive
Seek time	Depends on drive
Size	120mm D × 1.2mm
Cost	Depends upon disk and disk drive – DVD writers are still very expensive
Cost per 1MB	< £0.01
Advantages	Can store large amounts of data on the same size disk as a CD. Direct access.
Disadvantages	At the moment still expensive. Considered by some to be untested for medical applications.

Introduction

A DVD is essentially the same as a CD-ROM, but it utilises new technology to store more data on the same surface area. As technology advances more than ten times the information will be stored on the same size disks (see Chapter 13 – The Future).

Construction

This is the same as a CD-ROM, except that the size of the tracks that are encoded is very much smaller. The amount that a CD could store was limited by how close the track of the spiral could be without the laser misreading it. It was also limited by how small the bumps and troughs could be kept and still allow for accurate reading. Technology has improved enough for the data to be stored at a far higher density than was possible on a CD.

Read only DVDs utilise double layering, so instead of a single layer of pits and bumps there are two, with the outer one being covered with a thin coat of metal such as gold that a laser can focus through to read the layer underneath. This doubles the surface area for data to be stored. It is also possible to create a double-sided DVD that again doubles the total storage area of the DVD.

Acceptance of the audio CD was initially slow but is now fully accepted as the media for music at this present time. Familiarity with CDs has meant that the DVD has been very readily accepted into society and is likely to be a major storage media in the forthcoming years

Data Storage

Data is written in exactly the same way as a CD but utilising a finer wavelength laser that means that a finer tack can be created with smaller pits and bumps. As previously mentioned this means that more data can be stored.

DVD Readers

DVD readers again utilise the same technology as a CD-ROM reader, and DVD readers can read most CD formats but CD readers are unable to read DVDs.

Optical Disks

IN BRIEF

DAT	Optical Discs
Capacity	2.5GB+
Speed	CPU delivery rate
Seek time	Depends on drive – seconds
Size	Varies
Cost	£20.00
Cost per 1MB	< £0.01
Advantages	Tried technology
Disadvantages	Direct access. Difficult to correct data.

This is the more generic term for other optical disc recording systems that do not come under the other standards. They may be proprietary so it is important that the data being stored will be readable in the future. Optical disks have been utilised for a very long time, but the main problem with them has been the lack of any standards to ensure that one format has predominated over the rest.

They are of a similar construction to CD-ROMs but tend to be more robust because they come in a protective casing with a cover that is pulled back when the cassette is inserted into the reader (very similar to the floppy disk).

They tend to be double sided, but many readers will be single sided meaning that the disk has to be physically turned over to read the data on the other side. They can be incorporated into jukeboxes.

Magneto-optical disc systems

Magneto-optical systems utilise both a laser and a magnetic field to store data. The disk is made similar to a CD but the metallic surface within the disk has a uniform magnetic field applied across it. To write a bit of data a laser heats the material up to a critical point where the area under the laser is demagnetised. When it cools an applied magnetic field ensures that the area maintains a different magnetic field to the rest of the disc.

This area can be read by utilising a low powered polarised laser. The combination of laser and magnets allows for a very high density of data to be stored on the disc. These storage devices are also very robust.

Juke Boxes

Jukeboxes are devices that allow multiple archives of the same format to be available online without the need for a person to insert the appropriate disc or cassette. Having a jukebox reduces the cost of storage because cheaper technologies can be used, but it does increase the recall time as the archive that contains the requested image may take several minutes to come online.

However, flexibility is introduced into the system as more jukeboxes can be added as the archive increases with time or as new modalities are added.

VISUAL DISPLAY EQUIPMENT

MONITOR TECHNOLOGY

An understanding of monitor technology and monitor safety (discussed under Summary of Important Documents) is important as hospitals move towards the electronic record and a film-less hospital. It would perhaps seem necessary that each area where a film would have previously been viewed should be given the best quality monitor available, but this would be very expensive and most probably unnecessary.

Films are used for different purposes in different locations and the resolution required differs from location to location. It is however of vital importance that the differences in monitors are known in order that a decision can be made on the best visual display device for a specific location. Cost will also be an implication but should be secondary to the requirements of those who will be using the equipment to treat and diagnose.

TYPES OF MONITOR

There are basically two types of monitor, the traditional cathode ray tube (CRT) design and those that are put in the broad area of being 'flat screen' technologies.

Cathode Ray Tube

Basic Design

A CRT is a simple electron gun that via the process of thermionic emission emits electrons, which are drawn towards an anode via a potential difference. A stream of electrons is allowed through the anode and this stream of electrons is then focussed and steered using a magnetic coil. When the electrons collide with the crystals within the phosphor screen they impart their energy. The phosphor will emit light in the visible wavelengths, the intensity of which depends upon the intensity of the electrons colliding with it.

A black and white monitor is as simple as this with the tiny points of phosphor making up the visible image. Because the image is only made up of single points of light the image will be of a much higher resolution. White emitting phosphors are also capable of emitting far brighter light than colour monitors.

A colour monitor has three electron guns in order that three different phosphors (red, green and blue) can be stimulated at the same time. The other very different feature is the use of a shadow mask or an aperture grill to focus the electron beams onto the appropriate phosphor and to improve the image quality.

Shadow mask – this is a thin plate of metal placed just behind the phosphor with holes in it that match the circular phosphor elements. The electron beam is focussed through these holes

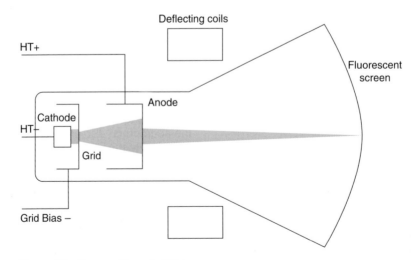

Figure 17 – Cross section of a CRT

to ensure that it hits the right phosphor every time.

Aperture Grill – this is made up of strips of very fine wire, which match strips of rectangular phosphor. This set up requires two supporting wires running horizontally across the grill and these can cause very faint artefacts on the screen.

Phosphors

In B&W systems the phosphor is a white light emitting phosphor. In colour systems the phosphors are red, green and blue, and are arranged in groups of three called triads. They can be made of either dots or stripes, depending on the system.

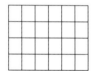

Figure 18 – Types of phosphor

Combinations of these colour phosphors can produce either an apparently grey scale image or a full colour image. CRTs take up a lot of space and the larger the dimensions of the screen the larger the length of the CRT behind it. CRTs also have a very large power consumption and these factors led to the development of flat screen technologies for the portable computer market. The benefits of these visual display devices are now available for static units at a reasonable price.

Flat Screen Monitors

Flat screen monitors are becoming more popular due to the minimal area that they take up but they are still very much more expensive than their CRT counterparts. There are many complex technologies that enable flat screen technology and only a brief overview will be given here.

Gas Plasma Display

Gas plasma displays are the oldest flat screen technology. They are created by constructing a matrix of tiny pixels of neon gas trapped between two electrodes. When the electrodes are turned on the gas glows. These systems have good contrast and resolution, but are limited to monochrome displays.

Liquid Crystal Displays

Liquid Crystal Displays (LCDs) work by utilising the unusual properties of liquid crystals. Liquid Crystals change shape when an electric current is passed through them. This can be utilised to either allow light to pass through the crystal or to prevent its passage. This can be used to turn an area black, as is the case in LCD digital watches and calculators.

The same technology can be used to act as a filter, varying the amount of red, green and blue light that is let through, thus allowing a full range of colours or grey scales to be displayed.

There are two types of LCD display:

Passive LCD Displays

Passive displays utilise a simple fluorescent light to the side of the screen and a reflective surface that directs the light out of the screen to be filtered by the LCD crystals. Passive displays tend to be dimmer and suffer from a certain amount of 'lag' in responding to a change in the screen environment.

They also have a narrow viewing angle. This means that the viewer must be seated directly in front of the screen to see the light coming from it. A television can be viewed from almost any angle because the light coming from the phosphors comes out from the surface in many directions. It is worth while trying this out on your television at home and comparing the viewing angles possible there with the viewing angles of other screens such as those found on laptops computers.

Active Displays

Active displays utilise light emitting diodes (LEDs) of red, green and blue under each pixel. These emit a much brighter light and they rival CRTs in contrast and resolution and also have a much larger viewing angle than passive displays. They are more expensive because of the more complex technology involved and because of the high failure rate during manufacture.

Factors Relating to Monitors

Dot Pitch

This refers to the resolution of the Screen, and is usually given in dots per inch (DPI) or dots per cm (DPC). It is measured from one colour to the next. This means that a black and white monitor is inherently sharper because the phosphor elements are much closer together. A monitor with a lower DPI will give a coarser image and may be hard to discern very small details on.

A typical PC monitor might be in the region of 90 DPI. A diagnostic grey scale monitor might be 171 DPI.

21–inch screen

This is the traditional measure of a screen, but this measure is perhaps now unsuitable for use in diagnostic imaging. The reason is that the majority of monitors were traditionally made to a 4/3 ratio, so rather than quote both dimensions the diagonal was given as the single figure that let you know the size of the monitor. However in diagnostic imaging monitors of different ratios are utilised for different purposes. A high-resolution monitor is generally capable of showing a full 35×43 in portrait format.

Because of the difference in the sizes of monitors used it is now common to give both the diagonal measurement and the number of pixels that can be demonstrated.

Resolution

This is the maximum number of pixels that the screen can demonstrate and is generally the same as the dot pitch. For a typical colour monitor this might be 1280×1024. For a high-resolution grey scale monitor this might be 2048×2560

This factor is important if you intend to display images at full resolution. For example the image that you want to display might be 2048×2048 matrix size. A 2048×2560 system would be able to display this at full size. A 1280×1024 would not be able to and up to four pixels at a time would have to be averaged to display the whole image.

This does not mean that it is unable to display the image at full resolution. It can display the image pixel for pixel, but only if the image is magnified. In this case approximately one quarter of the image would be visible at any one time

at full resolution. It is perfectly possible to show a high resolution image on a 64×64 matrix display device but so much of the image would not be visible that making a diagnosis would be nearly impossible. An important aspect of viewing an image is being able to look at the whole image as well as examining it in detail.

Luminance

Another factor quoted is the luminance of which the SI (system international) unit is the Candela. This is the recommended luminance that the system performs best at, and is an indication of how bright the image will be. Black and white monitors are inherently brighter.

Luminance is generally given for a certain distance, at which the apparent brightness is 1.

A colour monitor can be many times dimmer in luminance than its black and white counterpart.

Refresh Rate

This is the speed at which the electron beam(s) scan from the top to the bottom of the visible area. Monitors are typically in excess of 72 Hz, with televisions being less. Machines with lower refresh rates use interlacing to deceive the eye. If any flickering is visible then the refresh rate for the monitor is too low.

Colour Depth

This is the number of colours that your monitor is capable of showing. Usually given in bit depth.

Table 1 – Comparison of bit depth and available colours	
Bit Depth	**No of Colours**
1	2 – monochrome
2	4
4	16
8	256
16	65536 – high colour
24	16777216 – True colour

Footprint and Weight

These factors need to be considered, especially if the location of certain monitors may be in space limited areas (i.e. major trauma room). Also work surfaces must be tested to ensure that they can cope with the weight of the monitors.

Contrast layer

This is a layer that may be added to the front of the screen in order to absorb ambient light and allow for a much crisper image. This type of monitor is ideal for areas where there is poor ambient lighting but the coating will actually reduce the total luminance of the system.

Brightness and Contrast settings

These should be set to an acceptable level using a test pattern (SMPTE for example) and then locked into position. If different people are constantly adjusting them then none of the pre-programmed settings will be consistent and unnecessary changes to protocol may well be made. This may result in an increased dose to the patient. Manufacturers will detail the luminance that the system should be set to and this should be adhered to. (Further information is given under Chapter 9 – Image Quality).

Differences between Monitors and Televisions

Monitors tend to be smaller, have a higher resolution and each of the channels for the colours is controlled separately. Monitors also have faster refresh rate and often allow more user adjustment. A television, however, contains far more circuitry to receive and amplify the signal coming from the aerial cable. To display a television image a computer requires a specific adapter to convert the signal into a usable form for the monitor.

ACQUISITION TECHNOLOGIES

Every manufacturer has a slightly different system so the following is a guide based on one system. It will allow the reader enough knowledge to then understand how another manufacturers system differs and whether it will be able to perform the function required of it to an adequate level.

There are at the moment two clearly different technologies for acquiring digital images, computed radiography (CR) and digital radiography (DR and DDR).

COMPUTED RADIOGRAPHY EQUIPMENT

This essentially replaces the film with a recording phosphor that is read by a laser and the conventional processor with a workstation (and laser printer if required). It is very much like conventional radiography in appearance and use, and has a high acceptance amongst imaging staff. It is highly portable, with the cassettes weighing significantly less than conventional film screen combinations.

Its costs are certainly less than digital radiography systems, by virtue of the expense of the technology involved in digital radiography (see next section) and also has the advantage of being able to be incorporated into a departments current x-ray equipment. Many digital systems require the replacement of x-ray generating equipment as well as the recording and display media.

General Set Up

Here the equipment not covered in other sections will be explored. Figure 19 Shows the a typical set up for a computed radiography imaging system.

Cassette

This is a lightweight durable casing for the photo-stimulable phosphor. It does not have intensifying screens in, but it does have an anti-static material as the phosphor plates can store static electrical charges as artefacts on the image. The back is made of a thin sheet of aluminium to absorb x-rays. It is sealed when closed and easily cleanable. (Figure 20)

Phosphor Storage Plates

A phosphor plate looks to all intents and purposes like an intensifying screen. They are made of similar substances such as Europium activated Barium Fluoro-halide, and their construction is along the same lines, with an increased emphasis on protecting the screen from static electricity. This can be deposited within the plate or cause discharge of the signal stored there. Figure 21 shows basic phosphor storage plate construction.

The layers are composed of the following materials:

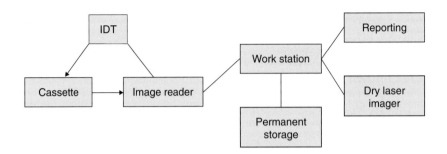

Figure 19 – General set up of a Fuji system

Figure 20 – Computed radiography cassette and phosphor

- Protective layer – thin and transparent to protect the phosphor.
- Phosphor – normally Barium Fluorohalide in a binder. This layer has colour centres that can be thought of as traps for electrons.
- Light shielding layer – sends light forward when released in the reader, ensuring as much light as possible is recorded. This will cause some unsharpness in the image.

- Conductive layer – removes static electricity and stray light.
- Support material – gives the plate strength
- Backing layer – soft polymer that protects the back of the cassette.

The above all have to provide a strong yet flexible plate that can endure hundred of transits into a reading device.

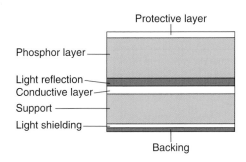

Figure 21 – Phosphor plate construction

There are both high resolution and fast phosphors with the high resolution have smaller phosphor crystals and a thinner phosphor layer which will of course require an increase in exposure to produce an acceptable image when compared to the fats phosphor. A typical system will have a 5 lp mm limiting resolution on an 18×24 cm plate and a 2.5 lp mm limiting resolution on a 35×43 imaging plate Phosphor stores the energy absorbed

Image Acquisition

The x-ray interacts with the electrons in the barium fluorohalide crystals, giving energy to them, which enables them to enter into the conduction band where they become trapped in what are called 'colour' centres. This is effectively the same as the latent image in conventional radiography.

Image Reading

In order to understand how the image is read it is important to have a basic understanding of how a laser works. In most systems the laser now used is a solid-state device, but the following explains how a traditional gas laser works which makes the principles easier to understand.

The LASER

Light normally comprises of many different wavelengths of light, often out of phase with each other. A laser is a device that emits a very coherent (in phase) beam of light in only one wavelength and that means that it contains a large amount of energy.

Laser stands for **L**ight **A**mplification of **S**timulated **E**mission of **R**adiation and each of these terms will be explained. In computed radiography this may be a solid-state laser or a neon helium gas laser.

When the power to the laser is turned on the neon atoms will be stimulated to emit light photons. These photons will interact with other atoms that are at a higher energy state because they are being given energy by the current flowing through the gas and atoms that are still at their ground state (low energy).

When half of the atoms are at the higher energy state **population inversion** is said to occur. Population Inversion is the point when the photons of light are more likely to interact

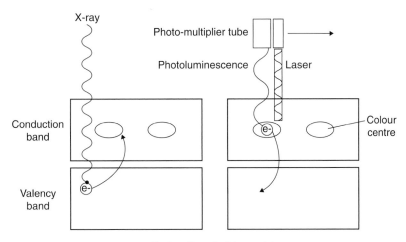

Figure 22 – Image plate acquisition and subsequent reading

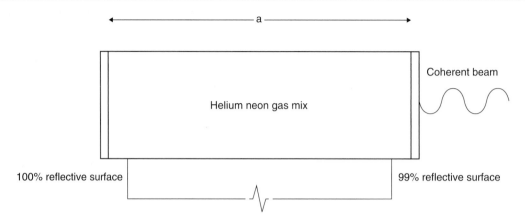

Figure 23 – Simple diagram of a continuous wave gas laser

with an atom in the higher energy state, as opposed to an atom still in its ground state (not excited).

The photon of light forces the excited atom back to its ground state, and in doing so the atom emits two photons of light and not the usual single photon. This is the Stimulated Emission of Radiation part of the process. The continuation of this process results in more and more light being emitted.

By using a 100% reflective surface opposite a 95–99% reflective surface the light can be bounced back and forth, causing more and more emissions of light by stimulated emission. This is the Light Amplification part. The distance between these reflective surfaces (a) precisely matches the wavelength of the photons of light and as they reflect back and forth they will end up in phase.

The small proportion of light photons that emerge through the partially reflective surface of the laser will be in phase, of the same wavelength and high in energy. This is the laser beam.

Image Reading Using a Laser

When the image plate is placed in the reader a helium neon laser scans the imaging plate in a simple non interlaced Rasta pattern (zig zag). This light comprises of a very narrow band of wavelengths. As it scans across the surface the laser imparts energy to any trapped electrons within the colour centres. With this extra energy the electrons are able to escape the colour cen-

tres and fall back to the valence band emitting excess energy in the form of visible light as they change energy levels.

The laser will scan across the plate again and again producing lines of intensity information (in a simple Rasta pattern). The light emitted is detected by a photo-multiplier, amplified and then the intensity digitised in an analogue to digital converter to be stored in the temporary memory. Once stored this signal may be automatically routed to a digital to analogue converter where it is then sent to a monitor or to a printer.

A problem with this system is that there are several areas for unsharpness to be introduced. Firstly when using any imaging plate made up of grains there will always be light scatter within the plate itself. This will result in unsharpness that is very similar to that found in intensifying screens (see figure 24)

Secondly there will be a finite distance between the surface of the phosphor plate and the photosensitive diode. This again allows for the light photons to spread out and unsharpness to be introduced (also shown on figure 24).

Image Erasure

As the image plate is scanned the electrons are all returned to the Valency band and this effectively removes the image from the plate. In case of accidental exposure the reader has a mode when it will scan the surface of the imager without recording the light emitted. This is its erasure mode. Other systems may automatically flood the

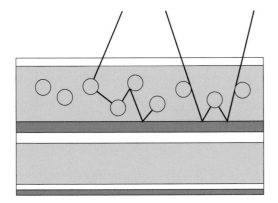

Figure 24 – Internal scatter external spread of light in a phosphor storage plate

plate with light to erase any electrons that are still trapped following the initial reading of the plate.

Phosphor storage plates are very sensitive to scatter and should be erased regularly to prevent the build up of any background signal. Some systems utilise a row of bright fluorescent lights that can remove any signal that has built up over time. See chapter on Image Quality and Quality Assurance for more details.

Summary of process
- The patient is x-rayed in the usual way, but the conventional film screen cassette is replaced with a phosphor storage plate cassette. This records the latent image.
- The IDT (identification terminal) is used to input the patient's details. The bar code reader then reads the image plate barcode so it knows which image plates are associated with which patient.
- At this point the computer is also told what view(s) has been done, e.g. wrist, CXR AP erect etc, which initialises the pre-set protocols for each image so that when they are finally displayed only minimal manipulation needs to be done (see image processing).
- The cassette is then taken to the image reader that is also connected to the IDT and knows which image plates are associated with which patients.
- The reader removes the plate from the cassette and then scans the image plate with a 100 μm laser. A photo-multiplier tube records the light that is then emitted by the crystals. The signal from this is amplified and sent to

the temporary storage via an Analogue to Digital Converter (ADC) and then to the monitor via a Digital to Analogue Converter (DAC).
- Permanent storage may be automatic or at the users control.
- User manipulation is possible at the workstation.
- Direct feedback on over/under exposure is visible via the sensitivity value (or other such parameter)
- Printing to hardcopy film is then possible (120 seconds approx).

DIGITAL RADIOGRAPHY

There are two types of systems, those that still produce an analogue signal (Indirect Digital Radiography) that subsequently has to be digitised and those that give a directly digital read out (Direct Digital Radiography).

The need for the traditional cassette and reader are removed and replaced by what is commonly called a flat panel detector (FPD). The patient is x-rayed on the detector, which automatically then sends the digital image to the temporary storage and then to the monitor. Detectors come in many forms, ranging from large fixed systems capable of imaging an area nearly 50cm^2, to small intra-oral devices that can provide digital dental radiographs.

This system necessitates the FPD to be connected to the image processor, normally by a cable. This has caused problems with mobile radiography where the cassettes must be entirely portable. FPDs do now exist with a built in memory that can be read when the cassette is returned to the department, but their construction makes them heavier than CR cassettes and potentially more fragile.

FLAT PANEL X-RAY IMAGE RECEPTORS CONSTRUCTION

There are two types of imaging receptor.

1 – Indirect Digital Imaging Receptor
The first type of detector is known as an indirect detector because the incoming x-rays are first converted to light photons before being detected. The basic construction of this type of flat panel detector (FPD) is shown in figure 26.

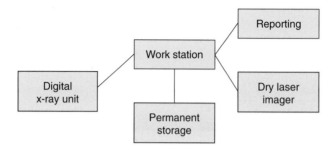

Figure 25 – Typical Digital Radiography Set-up

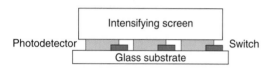

Figure 26 – Indirect image plate construction

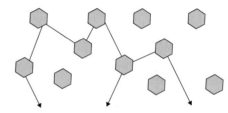

Figure 27 – Light scatter

The x-rays interact with the crystals in the intensifying screens and cause them to emit light. The photo-detector then detects the light photon and stores the intensity of the light in the form of an electrical charge proportional to the amount of light that fell on it. Each photo detector has a switch associated with it that is used to read out each of the elements of the plate in turn.

A problem with this type of device is the scattering of light within the phosphor, leading to a certain amount of unsharpness (figure 27). Intensifying screens have the same problems in this technology as they do in conventional radiography, i.e. light scatter and cross talk.

However the amount of unsharpness will be less than any unsharpness found in computed radiography systems. The signal that comes out of an indirect radiography device is said to be analogue because it takes the form of a gaussian curve (figure 28)

To create a charged coupled device (CCD) of the size required for a full chest x-ray is very expensive due to the large number of errors that are generated during manufacture. One solution is to have many smaller CCD areas that are

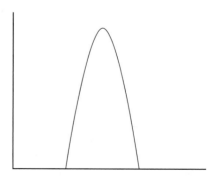

Figure 28 – Indirect Radiography output signal

placed next to each other. These areas are 'stitched' together to give what appears a seamless image.

There will be a slight decrease in resolution due to an increased 'dead' area between the CCD fields, but this will be imperceptible to the human eye.

A second method is to link the crystals to smaller CCD elements using optical cable to channel the light emitted. This makes for a more bulky cassette but does reduce the cost of the CCD elements. The same effect can also be produced using optics to focus the light onto the CCDs.

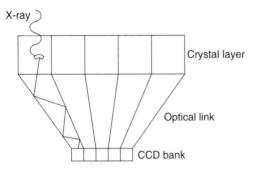

Figure 29 – Optically linked CCD

2 – Direct Digital Imaging Receptor

The second type of receptor is known as direct digital imaging. This uses crystals such as amorphous selenium, which directly converts the x-ray into electrical charge that is stored in a capacitor ready to be read. Again a switch is incorporated into the design to allow each of the elements to be read off (figure30)

The detector functions by placing a positive potential on the electrode in front of the Selenium. When an x-ray enters the selenium an

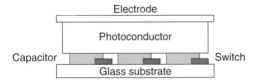

Figure 30 – Direct Radiography flat panel detector construction

electron and a positron are released. The electron is drawn towards the electrode, and the positron to the capacitor where it is stored to be read as electrical charge.

The benefits of this system are that there is zero scatter of the signal due to the columnar construction of the crystals that channel the charge to the appropriate receptor (figure 31)

The signal out looks much more like a square waveform (figure 32)

It is also said to be direct because there is no intermediate step, such as the light conversion that is present in the IDR system.

What has made both these technologies possible are active matrix liquid crystal displays (AMLCDs). This is the technology that allows the very thin lap top screens and now personal computer displays. The elements, switches and associated electrical connections are effectively built on top of the glass substrate. This process is expensive and has a high failure rate which leads to the high associated costs.

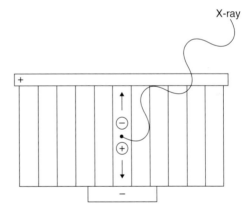

Figure 31 – Columnar construction of crystals

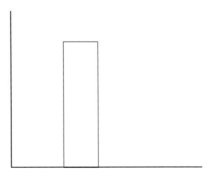

Figure 32 – Signal output from DDR

As previously mentioned there is a problem in making detectors of a suitable size. Smaller detectors can be made that are cheaper and more reliable, but this increases the amount of 'dead' space within an image. It also requires software to carry out a process known as 'stitching' to ensure a smooth image that looks as though it has been acquired as a whole.

The switches are normally constructed from thin film transistors (TFTs).

Image Reading

The imaging plate is made up of millions of these tiny detectors, typically in excess of 7,000,000 in an imaging plate 40cm × 40cm. Each of these tiny elements is not actually what will makes up the final pixel on an image (see image quality) but they can be thought of in this way. They are connected to amplifiers that enable the tiny signal that comes out of them to be boosted.

A charge equivalent to the number of light or x-ray photons received is stored in each element. A switching control organises the way in which the signals are read and thus the position that the signal came from (figure 33). This is then converted into the image.

Image Erasure

Once the switch is opened the photo-detector or the capacitor discharges completely, rendering it ready to receive another image.

Comparison of Two Systems

Both systems achieve a similar end but via very different routes. The differences can effectively be summarised under the following headings.

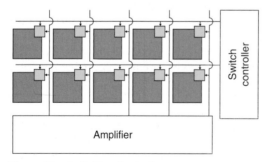

Figure 33 – Switching Control

- Cost
  CR is still very much cheaper than DR at the moment.

- Dose
  Similar minimal levels of dose reduction for both systems.

- Existing Equipment
  DR requires the replacement of existing equipment, whereas CR can simply replace current film screen and daylight processing systems.

- Resolution
  Comparable resolutions. CR should be higher by virtue it is recording data at a molecular level very similar to film, but the resolution is reduced by the laser size and unsharpness in the optical reading system.

- Speed
  DR is faster by virtue of the fact that there are no intermediate steps to delay the next image acquisition.

As systems proliferate the technology will become cheaper and more reliable. If the Electronic Patient Record is to become a reality then it is of vital importance that any new equipment installed within hospitals is one of the above. If it is not then the conventional system is likely to need replacing within a short space of time or some form of automatic digitisation will have to be undertaken.

Digital Scanners

A final and less satisfactory solution to producing digital images is to utilise a conventional film/screen combination and then scan the images subsequently. A scanner works by passing light through the radiograph and recording the intensity of light received at a photodiode or charge coupled device (CCD). Some scanners work utilising a single point of light that scans across the film in non-interlaced Rasta pattern. Others have multiple light sources and multiple detectors that allow a complete line to be scanned at a time, thus speeding up the process.

The larger the bank of detectors the more expensive the scanner will be, but the higher the possible throughput. Scanners can also be manual or automatic. Manual scanners require a user to physically put the film into the scanner and then tell the computer to begin scanning. An automatic scanner can take a pile of films and scan them without intervention. Scanners are available that fit directly onto the end of a daylight processor allowing automatic scanning of an image as it comes out of the processor.

All systems will, however, require a user to put the correct patient details with the correct image, which leaves the whole process open to errors. Scanned images will still require workstations to be displayed upon and extensive storage systems to deal with the data. Scanning can however be useful in building up a digital archive prior to moving over to a truly digital system.

Hardcopy Technologies

Introduction
There is no doubt that the ideal digital imaging system would completely remove hardcopy imaging from the equation and rely solely on softcopy transfer of information. This is unlikely to happen in the near future for several reasons.

- Poor proliferation of PACS within the current NHS
- Data size and subsequent transfer issues
- Display technology limitations
- User acceptance issues

These reasons mean that hardcopy devices are likely to remain a part of radiography for some time. This section will give a brief explanation of the types of printers that may be found in current use. Some have been in used for some time and others are relatively new and have been designed with the digital imaging market in mind.

Wet Processing Techniques
Many departments are still utilising daylight wet processing systems that utilise chemicals to develop the latent image on the film. There are both health and safety issues and environmental issues surrounding the use of such chemicals and the current trend is to move away from wet processing and towards dry processing technologies.

Video Hardcopy Units
These utilise a small cathode ray tube that displays the image that is to be copied. A sheet of single emulsion x-ray film is exposed to the light and subsequently processed. These types of imaging devices are typically low resolution and prone to image artefacts. They were popular in ultrasound, nuclear medicine and mobile image intensifiers due to their low cost.

Laser Printers
These systems were first developed for the computed tomography (CT) market to allow fast, variable image layout printing. In the same way as a television scans the phosphor screen in a raster pattern the laser would scan the film. Once processed a very high quality image resulted. The benefits of this system were the variable number of images that could be displayed on a single sheet of film, the high quality and larger throughput (90 second processing with the subsequent film only being 30 seconds behind the previous film). The main disadvantage was that the system still utilised wet processing with the associated chemicals and environmental issues.

Dry Processing Techniques
Introduction
These systems utilise no wet chemicals making them easy to install and environmentally friendly. Whilst approaching the quality of wet processed films they lack the maximum density achievable using conventional wet processing systems.

Photo-thermographic Printing
This utilises a laser to scan the image onto the film in the same way as a conventional laser imager, but the film contains all of the processing chemicals within its emulsion. Once through the laser the film is exposed to a thermal head that activates the chemicals and develops the image. The chemicals remain in the film.

Thermographic Printing
This uses heat to directly cause a change in the silver behenate within the film thus exposing and developing the film at the same time. This technology is very reliable, although not quick. It also has the added advantage of allowing the film to be opened and reloaded in daylight without fogging the film.

Microcapsule is a variation of this where the film contains capsules that are made permeable to the surrounding developing agent within the film when exposed to heat. This will turn an area of the film black, which becomes permanent once cooled.

An issue with all thermal imaging techniques is that if they are subsequently exposed to heat artefacts can be introduced. This means that the films do need to be handled and stored carefully.

Other Printing Techniques

There are also several other techniques that are at the moment more traditionally used for text printing, but there is little reason that they could not be used in some aspect of medical imaging. At the moment the convention is still to produce an image that requires light to be transmitted through it to view it (i.e. from a light box). This may change as those using the technology become used to viewing images in different ways.

Conventional Laser Printer

This type of laser printer scans the image onto a rotating drum that becomes charged wherever the laser hits it. The drum rotates through a toner that becomes attracted to the charged portion of the drum. The toner is then transferred to the paper via heat and pressure resulting in the printed image. This is the same technology that modern photocopiers use.

Dye Sublimation

These printers utilise a thermal head to release the dye directly onto the paper, which results in a very high contrast image. Often used for printing textual information and barcodes.

Inkjet Printer

These are currently the most common form of printer and utilise ionised ink that is sprayed onto the paper utilising magnetic fields. These are very inexpensive but their overall speed is slow and the resolution is low.

REFERENCES AND SOURCES

BOOKS

Boden L 1995 **Mastering CD-ROM technology** John Wiley and Sons

Byrd W 1995 **Understanding Computers** Jain Publishing Company

Carlton R.R., Adler A.M. 1996 **Principles of Radiographic Imaging** Delmar Publishers, London

Carter P.H. 1994 **Chesney's Equipment for Student Radiographers** Blackwell Scientific Publications, London

Davies A., Fennessy P. 1994 **Electronic Imaging for Photographers** Focal Press, Oxford

Davies A., Fennessy P. 1998 **Digital Imaging for Photographers** Focal Press, Oxford

Doi K., Macmahon H., Giger M.L., Hoffman K.R. 1998 **Computer-Aided Diagnosis in Medical Imaging** Elsevier, Amsterdam

Gonzalez R.C., Woods R.E. 1992 Digital Image Processing Addison Wesley Publishing Wokingham

Graham R. 1998 **Digital Imaging** Whittles Publishing, Scotland

Greenfield G.B., Hubbard L.B. 1984 **Computers in Radiology** Churchill Livingstone, London

Gunn C. 1994 **Radiographic Imaging** Churchill Livingstone, London

Hajnal J.V., Hill D.L.G., Hawkes D.J. (eds) 2001 **Medical Image Registration** CRC Press, London

Kuni C.C. 1988 **Introduction to Computers and Digital Processing in Medical Imaging** Year Book Medical Publishers, London

Pizzutiello R.J. (ed) 1993 **Introduction to Medical Radiographic Imaging** Eastman Kodak Company, New York

Robertson I 1995 **Hard Drives Made Simple** Butterworth Heinemann Ltd

Russ J.C. 1998 **The Image Processing Handbook** CRC Press, London

Watteville A de, Naughton S 1998 **Advanced Information Technology** Heinemann

Wilson B 1996 **Information Technology: The Basics** Macmillan

WWW

http://www.life.rmit.edu.au/mrs/ DigitalRadiography/
Excellent resource with many links.

http://www.hologic.com/prod-dr/ tech-directray.shtml
Direct radiography site

http://www.sunnybrook.utoronto.ca:8080/
~selenium/basics.html
>   Indirect and direct radiography acquisition
    technologies

http://www.usa.canon.com/indtech/medeq/
drs.html
>   Examples of equipment and applications
    from Canon

http://www.odont.au.dk/rad/Digitalx.htm
>   Large number of links for digital dental
    radiography

http://www.diagnosticimaging.com/
>   The online magazine with much information

4: INTERFACE STANDARDS

Terry Jones & Jason Oakley

INTRODUCTION

As mentioned in previous chapters, the secret to a storage media lasting is the setting of a clearly defined standard that will allow the device to be read by machines made by multiple manufacturers. The most graphic example of this was the extensive standard initially set for the Video Home System (VHS) tape.

Despite the Betamax tape having higher specifications, VHS soon predominated the market. This was because the standard allowed multiple manufacturers to create both their own tapes that could be read in other manufacturers tape players and their own tape players, which could play a variety of other manufacturers tapes.

Before any digital equipment was developed few such standards existed in radiography, and a manufacturers processing system was designed to be used with a specific film screen combination. Mixing and matching of systems was possible through trial and error, but they were not designed to be interchangeable and nobody thought seriously about doing this.

With the advent of the first digital imaging device, the Computed Tomography (CT) scanner, came the possibility of storing information in a new way, namely digitally. This could be done in one of many formats including the manufacturers own. At this time there was only the beginning of the concept that this data might need to be transferred between machines, and this lead to many machines writing data in what has become known as proprietary format.

CT scanners are still in existence that are storing information in this format and the problem is that once the scanner is replaced the data that has been stored cannot be easily be read by other devices. An interface could be designed, but such custom made devices are not always reliable and can also be very expensive.

However, the manufacturers did realise that this problem was going to occur as more and more modalities developed digital solutions. This stimulated the idea of a taking the images from an acquisition device such as CT, and reviewing them at remote locations, the first form of teleradiology. From this came the concept of the filmless hospital with all of the images from all of the imaging modalities potentially being shared amongst hospital wide and eventually nationwide professionals.

For this to happen a standard format for images and information within hospitals had to be developed, but due to the complex nature of this data this could not be done overnight.

This chapter will look at two standards that have come to dominate within hospitals in the United Kingdom over the last twenty years, Digital Imaging and Communication in Medicine (DICOM) and Health Level 7 (HL7). These two standards are very extensive and could easily warrant a book to themselves. The focus of this chapter will be to give the reader a good understanding of what the standards attempt to achieve and the way in which they achieve it.

Because DICOM is the predominant standard used at the moment for digital imaging in radiology this will be focussed on. HL7 was initially a standard for textual information within hospitals and DICOM the standard for images, but both standards are now moving beyond their initial limitations to encompass all information within hospitals and thus provide a single standard.

This may lead to the situation where by all information within a single hospital is compatible but information between hospitals is not. This is one of the areas that the NHS Information Authority (NHSIA) is attempting to address. Such organisations are not concerned with how something is done; they are there to make sure that it is done appropriately. Their guidance does not set out to say which software should be used, or what format the information should be in, but states what that software or standard must be able to do to allow for the electronic record to become a reality.

This should ensure that no matter what standard is being used the information is easily available to all those that require access to it and that expensive interfaces are avoided.

GENERAL CONSIDERATIONS FOR STANDARDS

There are several generic issues that standards must address and these are not difficult concepts, but are areas that should be of the utmost importance.

Connectivity – systems must be able to connect with other systems, utilising an interface device if necessary, but ideally on a system to system connection. This is an important consideration when setting up stand-alone temporary systems. The future proofing of connectivity will ensure that the system can connect into a larger network at a later date.

One way to ensure this is to make sure that any system being purchased adheres to recognised standards and can also prove that they can connect with other systems. The Radiological Society of North America's (RSNA) annual meeting has demonstrated this many times in the last few years, setting up virtual hospitals where multiple vendors can demonstrate how their systems are capable of interfacing.

Reliability or robustness – This has two distinct facets. Firstly the integrity of the image or data following transfer from one system to another must be without question. Secondly the way that the system deals with component failures to prevent loss of patient information must also be evaluated.

Security – the systems must be able to prevent access by unauthorised persons or viruses that might result in the loss of patient data. All security should be multi level and controlled by a single person who is responsible for the overall security of the system. The integrity of the security of the system may come under close scrutiny in future medico-legal cases.

DATA COMPONENTS

In order to understand what the standards attempt to achieve it is necessary to first understand the various components of a digital medical image file. This will be very similar to a file dealing just with patient data.

Figure 1 depicts the parts of an image that can easily be differentiated, but are taken for granted as being part of the image. The first part is normally termed the header and this contains many important pieces of information such the patients name, the type of image, the matrix size etc. It is this part that tells a program trying to read the file whether it can in fact read it and what the various components of it are. The final part of the file, which may be the largest part, is the data of the actual image itself, the binary code that tells the program reading it which grey scale or colour should be present in a certain position on the image.

These two key components are still used in all standards, but it is the way they are laid out and read that ensures that the files are compatible between different systems.

DICOM

There are many terms that are peculiar only to DICOM so an accessory glossary has been included at the beginning of this section to aid the readers understanding.

> Attribute (in DICOM) – A property of an Information Object. An attribute has a name and value which are independent of any encoding scheme.

Header

Name
DOB
Images
Modality
Matrix

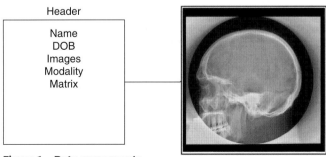

Figure 1 – Data components

AE Title − Application Entity Title. A DICOM term used to distinguish a piece of equipment on a network. Along with an IP address this makes the equipment unique on any network and allows DICOM equipment to recognise and communicate with each other

CR − Computed Radiography

DICOM − Digital Image Communication in Medicine

DMWL − DICOM Modality Worklist. A method of obtaining patient demographics direct from your RIS onto your modality without the need for typing

MRI − Magnetic Resonance Imaging

Q/R (Query Retrieve) − A DICOM term used to explain the function of sending a patient query from one DICOM device to another. Both units must agree they know each other (DICOM association) before the images are allowed to be released. Q/R is slower than a simple DICOM send

RIS − Radiology information system.

SCP − Service class provider (e.g. image store)

SCU − Service class user (e.g. sender)

SOP − Service Object Pair (SCU and SCP)

This section will also refer to compression as a potential tool within DICOM. This is discussed more fully in Chapter 8 − Image Processing but there are two terms that it is important to understand. Lossless compression refers to a reduction in the size of the storage requirement of the image with no loss of quality. Lossey compression refers to a larger reduction in the storage requirement of the image with a loss in image quality. With lossey compression, there may or may not be a reduction in the diagnostic usefulness of the image. As always, tests should be performed on any compression to assess the suitabilty of that image for its intended purpose.

History of DICOM

In view of the need for an international standard for digital medical images the National Electrical Manufacturers Association (NEMA), in associa-tion with the American College of Radiologists (ACR) set out in the early 1980s to produce a standard that multiple manufactures could adhere to, allowing communication between medical imaging equipment from different man-ufacturers.

The first standard, known as ACR-NEMA, began development in 1982 and was first avail-able in 1985 and dealt with very basic elements of point-to-point transfer of images to ensure that when the destination system displayed the image it was displayed identically to the original.

Version two was released in 1988 with many enhancements to the original standard, and this should give the reader an idea of the problems involved in developing a standard and the asso-ciated time scales involved. However, every modification of the standard was an improve-ment. Another reason that the standard was constantly being revised was that other modali-ties were becoming digital and thus had to be incorporated into the standard.

In addition to this modalities were also advancing, producing new ways of acquiring and displaying information and this too had to be added to the standard. This process is still going on today; best exemplified in the change in CT acquisition methods, firstly to helical and then to multi-slice helical, each step presenting new challenges to the DICOM standard. DICOM also has to be able to cope with the ever-expanding roles of MRI and Ultrasound.

With the advent of networking a large change in the standard was required and to highlight this it was given a new name, DICOM.

The process has been a slow one and is con-tinuing, but the standard has already evolved into the far more reaching DICOM 3.0 standard that exists today. DICOM is still not complete. It is being modified all of the time as emerging tech-nologies reveal issues of communication that had not previously been considered.

DICOM is by no means a global standard, although due to the international nature of the companies involved it has been discussed or parts of it used in many other standards. It remains to be seen which standard will eventu-ally dominate.

Definition

DICOM is a set of instructions (standards) to manufacturer's that allows different modalities within radiology (or medicine if images are involved) to communicate with each other. It is now being expanded to set a standard for all information within hospitals.

DICOM is not a file format (like bitmap – *.BMP or JPEG – *.JPG), but a set of standards that describe a file format.

DICOM strives to remove the problems that can occur when different manufacturers use different protocols in their systems, without taking away the manufacturers ability to include a factor that makes their equipment unique. This is important because it is the uniqueness of a piece of equipment that not only sells it, but also drives the technology forward.

DICOM and Field Contents

In file formats prior to DICOM, all of the information required by other systems was present but not in a form that the other system could recognise. As an example, a computer is able to interpret text if it is in a format that it is programmed to deal with:

John Doe m 010170 123456789 Admitted E4 010102

However, a computer is unable to discern that these different groups of characters have any meaning. For an individual system, the computer might be programmed to be aware that the first part of the information was the patient's name, the second the patient's sex, the third the date of birth and so on. However, another system might expect the date of birth first, followed by the patient's unique identifier.

Image attributes are also stored in the same way. Many systems, in order to reduce the memory requirement of an image, do not store the x-y co-ordinates of the individual pixels of an image, but instead store a continuous line of grey scale values as though the image had been stretched into a single line. All the computer needs to reconstruct this image is the matrix size into which this string of data needs to fit. Without this the image will be unintelligible.

The list of additional information that could be sent with the image, and in many cases is important for the image to be used diagnostically, can be very long. With the advent of volume acquisitions in CT and MRI it is vitally important that the information is easily available to allow processing of the data sets on powerful workstations.

DICOM attempts to provide a level playing field where every one knows the rules in order that at a basic level one system can communicate with another system. The manufacturers also know what they are allowed to do outside of this in order to allow developments in technology. It is also accepted that as technology changes new fields that were once 'private' may become compulsory to allow exchange of information.

The use of 'fields' allows lots of information to be attached to an image and guarantee that another system can effectively read it. Every hospital will have a unique identifier that sits in a specific field. Every modality has a unique identifier that again sits in a specific field. There will be a field for the patients surname, forename, date of birth etc.

DICOM and Information Exchange

As well as determining what information a file contains and where it should contain it DICOM also governs the way in which information exchange takes place. For the exchange of information to take place a number of things need to be present

Application Entity Title (AET)

Each component of a system such as a CT scanner will have its own AET. Along with the unique identifier for the hospital (which is globally unique) this gives every image taken in the world a unique identifier. All components of the system are programmed with an AE List (AEL). This is a list of other computers that they are allowed to exchange information with.

Service Object

This is the part of DICOM that lists what the actual modality is, such as CT or MRI, permanent storage etc.

Service Class

Examples of these classes include

- Storage
- Query
- Retrieval

Service classes define what a system is able to do, such as store images, retrieve images or print images. If a system has not been set up with a certain class, it will be unable to perform that task. It is this part of DICOM that is used to attempt to connect with another system to establish if they are able to carry out the required function.

Within the service class there will also be specific services. An example of this under Storage would be Store CT images. A CT scanner that wishes to store images can only use this DICOM service application if the system it is attempting to store to also has the appropriate service class set up. A system can claim to be DICOM compliant even if it is only able to perform one of these services within a service class.

This means that a system that claims to be DICOM compatible, that only supports printing cannot communicate with another system, that is also DICOM compatible, but for the storage component.

In DICOM each piece of equipment is labelled as either a Service class user (SCU) or a service class provider (SCP). It is also possible for a system to be labelled as both.

As an example we will look at storage as the service that is being used at this time.

A DICOM SCU piece of equipment will act as a sender of information of the TYPE that equipment belongs too. This in essence is the modality. Hence a modality that supports a CR SCU is not able to send an image taken on a DICOM MRI scanner (unless the equipment also has an SCU component for MRI).

Most PACS archives have a DICOM SCP for ALL modalities that are likely to be sending images to it. If a PACS does not have a SCP component for Nuclear Medicine (for instance) then it will not be able to deal with those images. Some PACS can allow storage of any image, but if they do not have the DICOM component they are unable to deal with the images in a meaningful way.

So a system that creates a DICOM image has been set up to produce an image using the DICOM standard, but DICOM is not in itself a file format. Adherence to this standard allows the image to be used by the service classes set up on different systems in a reliable manner.

Information objects

The information to be stored can be broken down into groups of related information known as information objects. These give structure to the information that the DICOM file contains. An Information object contains information on

what are termed the 'real world' properties of the image, such as patient details.

Each information object, such as the object containing patient details, has areas into which information must go, such as forename, surname etc. Even if the information is not present the object maintains its structure. So each information object class definition consists of a description of the objects purpose (i.e. to contain patient details) and also a description of the attributes that it contains (forename etc).

However the breaking down of information into distinct objects or information entities does have a disadvantage. Many of the objects within DICOM need to be seen together, or as multiple information entities to make any sense. For this reason objects are either termed normalized (they mean something on their own) or composite (required to be read in conjunction with other information entities because they are part of the image information).

Normalised

This contains information that can mean something in its own right and is made up of only one set of data (information entity). An example would be the patient information object, which contains simply patient information. This can be made sense of on its own, although may be of minimal use.

Composite

Composite objects are called this because they are made up of more than one information entity. As an example an MRI image would be made up of patient details, study details, equipment details and the image itself. Because it is made of more than on information entity it is known as composite.

A composite image may contain information that could be normalised, but the other files require that information to ensure that the image is of maximum use.

DICOM Message Service Elements (DIMSE's)

Because there are two types of information objects there needs to be two set of instructions to allow systems to carry out functions on the data. These can be either DIMSE-N or DIMSE-C for the normalised or composite information objects. There are 5 DIMSE-C are 6 DIMSE-N.

DIMSI-C
Store
Get
Find
Move
Echo

DIMSE-N
Create
Set
Get
Delete
Action

Event Report
This simple set of instructions is used to make up the more complex functions that are known as the service classes and are used to manage the information through the use of the aforementioned service object pairs (SOPs).

DICOM and Compression
DICOM does support the lossless compression of images and goes on to define several different levels of JPEG compression. Just as it is important to ensure that systems that are required to communicate have matching service classes, it is equally important that compression capabilities are also matched.

DICOM Modality Work List (DMWL)
A useful function of any system is the ability to be able to collate which patients will be going to which piece of equipment for any given day. This prevent errors from the re-inputting of data (typing) at the modality and frees up time to do other tasks. DICOM has a built in ability to do this.

Problems with DICOM
There is little doubt that there is a vast difference in the level to which manufacturers support DICOM because the standard is open to interpretation. As problems arise the DICOM standard is tightened up to ensure that the same issues do not rise again.

So the basics of what the DICOM standard achieves is to provide known fields into which information can be stored, retrieved, acted upon and forwarded between systems. It is not at this time perfect, but it has gone a long way to creating the seamlessly interfacing systems that is the over all goal of such standards.

HL7

The international standard for communication of electronic data is the International Standards Organisation's (ISO) Operating Systems Interconnect (OSI). This was the ISO's attempt to ensure that all systems could interconnect freely. However, many of the parameters were loosely defined so it is not considered totally reliable.

OSI set out to achieve a number of things;

- Allow the transmission of data across a physical medium
- Route data to the correct location
- Be able to recognise data
- Be able to check data
- Allow the interaction with a user

It works via a system of seven layers to make sure that transmission is as efficient as possible (See Summary of Important Documents).

Health Level 7 sought to further refine the seventh level of this standard (Applications) for healthcare use, and thus the standard was defined as Health Level Seven. As previously mentioned the initial aim was to set a standard for textual information.

The standard was developed over a period of time by meetings between multiple vendors and users. This demonstrates an important principle that should be seen more in the development of information technology for the health service; the consultation of those who will be using the system on what they want it to do and how they want it to do it.

It was considered important to have a standard because of the previous unreliability of transfer of data between systems that could potentially lead to a misdiagnosis or administration of the wrong treatment.

The aim was to make it easier for systems from different manufacturers to interface, and ideally remove the need for a complex interface. The chapter on networks states that PACS comes alive when it interfaces with other systems. In the same way a stand-alone hospital information system (HIS) is useful on its own, but when it can communicate freely with a radiology information system (RIS) they can be of far more use.

The HIS can update the RIS automatically as patient data changes, and if desired any changes can also go from the RIS to the HIS. Events within RIS can also trigger events in the HIS and vice versa, meaning that all systems within the hospital are aware of what is happening to a specific patient, helping to prevent mistakes being made.

HL7 was extremely ambitious because it set out to provide a standard that could be used by all text based information systems within a health care environment, regardless of whether they were clinical or not. The same standard would apply for the financial services within the hospital as to information coming from the pathology laboratory or from the laundry services department. As was to be expected there were many manufacturers producing equipment for specific purposes, and thus the standard has taken some time to be accepted.

A patient's pathway through the hospital and the number of events that can be attributed to that patient are also large and thus the standard was not just for the transfer of that information but the event triggered transmission of data. The philosophy was that rather than an individual having to seek out information every time a patient presented to them, the information would already have been prepared and sent because it would have been triggered by the patient's admission or out patient's appointment etc.

This is possible because the majority of the information will be in the form of text and this ensures that the information can not only be read by a subsequent system but can also be used for other purposes.

The way in which HL7 does this is to ensure that the information is encoded in such a way that subsequent computers will know what the fields mean. A string of text in a standard format can be read by any computer but it will not mean anything to it and it will not be able to identify specific fields. For example:

John Doe m 010170 123456789 Admitted E4 010102

This string of text contains much information and we, as humans, can extract information from it because we are able to make suppositions about what the data means. However a computer can do no such thing. The computer has to be told what each of the field means. To do this HL7 breaks up a message into distinct segments.

Message Header Segment
All transmitted files have a header that will contain similar information. The message header in HL7 contains the source of the information plus the destination and time relevant details. So in our example the data might come from the HIS and be going to the RIS in case the patient requires diagnostic imaging.

Event Type Segment
This field is determined by specific codes that refer to patient events such as patient transfer, discharge etc In this case the patient is being admitted and the location of the admission is E4. Codes are used for each potential event.

Patient Identification Segment
This would identify the patients name, DOB, hospital number etc. and each of these fields would be separately identified to ensure no confusion. In our example the computer would have to be made aware that the surname is Doe, the first name is John, the date of birth is 1st January 1970, sex Male and unique identifier 123456789.

There are many other segments and codes that might be used. In order to define them specific separators are used to let the system know that a new segment or component of a segment is next.

For non HL7 devices a purpose built interface engine can be used to convert the data to HL7 format which can then be subsequently transferred to all other HL7 compliant systems. In the same way that being DICOM compliant does not mean that a system is compliant in all areas it is possible for a system to claim to be HL7 compliant and actually require some degree of patching or translation to enable a true connection to be made.

HL7 is not a global standard, but in the US in the region of 90% of large hospitals are utilising it as much as possible. It again is not a fixed standard but is growing all of the time to encompass new tasks that are being created and to ensure that current fields are adequate for the uses to which they are being put.

Some of HL7 was used as the basis of textual information storage in the DICOM standard.

IHE

Integrating Health Enterprise

Current estimates indicate that approximately 30% of the cost of any PACS installation will be spent on integration; that is getting systems to talk efficiently. This is despite the use of standards such as DICOM and HL7. Integration is therefore costly to the purchaser in terms of money, but it is also costly to the vendor in terms of the time and effort that it can take to get a system to do all of the things that it is supposed to.

The IHE sought to increase the users perception of manufacturers solutions to digital healthcare by involving them in the thought and design processes. This enables the manufacturers to give the users what they actually want, not what the manufacturers think they should have.

As well as the users the IHE has strived to bring together manufacturers from all areas of healthcare, including those out side of DICOM and medical imaging, such as HL7, to ensure that they can seamlessly be interfaced. The ultimate aim would be for health care systems to be as near to the personal computer ideal of 'plug and play' as possible.

This increases the efficiency of information technology within the healthcare environment and at the same time makes the installation of equipment easier for the manufacturers. The ability to interface easily also means that during procurement the project manager can focus only on those pieces of equipment that are able to this. Market forces will mean that more manufacturers will strive for this standard and the increase in vendors in the market place will improve prices.

CONCLUSIONS

Standards are an essential part of the future of information technology in the NHS, but a standard is difficult to write, and even more difficult to implement. For this reason no one standard is global at this time, and it will be some years before a truly global solution to the transfer of image data is settled upon.

During procurement it is the setting up of the interface between systems that ensures that the overall performance of the system is as desired. Changing the systems capabilities belatedly will be time consuming and costly and should be avoided at all costs.

SOURCES

www.xray.hmc.psu.edu
   Many DICOM Resources

http://medical.nema.org/
   Official DICOM home page

http://www.hl7.org/
   Official HL7 home page

www.rsna.org
   Radiological Society of North America

http://www.hl7.org.uk/
   UK affiliated web site for HL7

http://www.rsna.org/IHE/index.shtml
   Official IHE Home page

http://www.rsna.org/REG/practiceres/dicom/nontechintro.html
   A non-technical introduction to DICOM

http://www-pet.umds.ac.uk/~eds/dicom.html
   Basic DICOM introduction

http://www.psychology.nottingham.ac.uk/staff/cr1/dicom.html
   Basic DICOM introduction

http://www.dominator.com/customertools/dicom.htm
   An introduction with some detail on DICOM

http://www.expresshealthcaremgmt.com/20001216/medsoft1.htm
   Excellent introduction to DICOM

http://www.rsna.org/REG/practiceres/dicom/services.html
   RSNA non-technical introduction to DICOM

5: NETWORKING AND INTERFACING

Marco Crispini

Interfacing is what makes PACS come alive. When you metaphorically take your brand new PACS out of its box, of course the visual bits are initially the most exciting – being able to window width and level, to zoom in, and to play generally. But the rewards from a fully interfaced PACS continue beyond the initial unwrapping. As you find each new way of working, each incremental improvement, you realise that interfacing is what makes PACS *really* useful.

But before we discuss the data and desired effects of interfacing, I will give an overview of how these systems may be physically interconnected, namely the network, and explain in plain language key networking jargon. However, this is not a pre-requisite to understanding interfacing, and the reader is invited to jump straight to interfacing if so desired.

NETWORKING

A network is in essence the physical wires that connect two or more systems. A single piece of wire can be a network if only two systems are connected. For a real-world network with more than two systems, more wires as well as specialised pieces of equipment are required. Surprisingly for an industry so full of jargon, these pieces of equipment are called *network equipment*.

The "wires" that comprise a network may also be fibre optic or even radio waves in the case *wireless networks*. But for simplicity, we will still think of them as copper wires or *cables*.

Just as you can communicate face to face, over the telephone, by letter, email or via a lawyer, there are different ways that a network can be set up. In addition, a network may be one of a few different types, just as your communications may be in English, French or Japanese. The most common types, or *protocols*, are *Ethernet, token ring,* and *ATM*.

All of these things add complexity – more functions and more pieces of equipment to perform them – and therefore more jargon. But the concept is still simple – to allow one system to communicate with another.

NETWORK SPEEDS

Electricity passing along the wires is the information and images that the network is carrying – a low voltage representing 1, and zero volts representing 0. Everything including electricity takes time to get from A to B. Even light, which travels so fast man took thousands of years to realise it even travels at all, takes a now measurable amount of time to get from A to B. But for networks at least think of the travel from A to B as instantaneous. Just like when the mains electricity is switched on to your home – it "instantly" appears at every single socket.

So what limits the speeds of networks? The 1 or 0 must *definitely* be recognised as a 1 or 0. You would miss a light if it was switched on for only 1/1000th of a second – you would need perhaps a ¼ or a ½ second to definitely say "the light came on, so that represents a 1." This is the same with network equipment and the part of the computer systems that the wires plug into – called the *network card*, or less commonly *NIC* or *network interface card*.

Each 1 or 0 is called a *bit*, and network speeds are measured in millions of bits per second, or *megabits per second* (*Mb/s*). Do not confuse network speeds with the measure of memory and disk capacity, which is *bytes, megabytes* (*Mb*), or *gigabytes* (*Gb*).

Interference in our imperfect world also limits speeds. Imagine a slight flicker in the light bulb. If we have a ½ second representing 1 then a slight flicker is irrelevant. But as we try to use a shorter and shorter time to represent 1, it becomes increasingly difficult to differentiate between flicker and genuine signal. So the quality of the wires is very important too.

Category 3 UTP cable for example can run at up to 10Mb/s. *Category 5 UTP* cable can run at up to 100Mb/s. UTP cables are the network cables that look like they have a telephone jack at each end. The category numbers are arbitrary, other than a higher number indicating a higher maximum speed. Knowing the UTP acronym doesn't help us day to day nor in our understanding. Just use the term "UTP." But for the record it's *unshielded twisted pair*.

To take advantage of *"Cat 5,"* as category 5 UTP is often contracted to, you also need 100Mb/s network cards in each computer system. Intermediate network equipment, if any, must also run at 100Mb/s or higher.

These speeds sound fast but the average CR chest is 6 to 8Mb (mega*bytes*) and each byte is eight bits so you don't need many people working at the same time before you reach maximum capacity.

Bandwidth is the amount of capacity available to transfer information. A network running at a speed of 100Mb/s has ten times the bandwidth, or capacity, of a 10Mb/s network. Of course, if many pieces of equipment share a network, then this sharing reduces the amount of bandwidth available to each individual piece of equipment.

ETHERNET, NODES AND IP ADDRESSES

Ethernet is the most common protocol today. It is the protocol the Internet uses, which explains why some of its terms are so common, for example *IP address*. An IP address is literally an address, so information can get to its intended destination. It takes the form of 4 numbers, separated by dots, e.g. 192.55.1.121, and must be unique. Another completely separate network could use the same IP address, but only so long as the two networks are never connected. Every *node* on the network is given a unique IP address. A node is any piece of equipment that communicates on the network. A computer system (e.g. your PC) is the most common node, but it could be a printer, a piece of network equipment, a CT scanner, etc. Nowadays even personal stereos can be a node, allocated an IP address and plugged into a network to download music.

SENDING IMAGES

Imagine a network with 3 nodes:

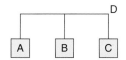

Figure 1

If A is a CT scanner (or more precisely the CT scanner's workstation) and it wants to send a scan to the PACS server, C, it writes the information onto the network. The low voltage signals "instantly" appear at all nodes on the network, in this case just B and C. Both read the *header*, the first part of any information sent across the network. The header includes the destination IP address. B sees the information isn't addressed to B and discards the information; C sees that the information is, and reads the CT scan.

COLLISIONS

Now imagine that B is a computer that attempts to write to the network at the same time that A starts sending its CT scan. The two sets of signals interfere with each other making both sets unintelligible. A *collision* has occurred. This is detected and both nodes wait for a short while and then retry. This short delay varies randomly so that both nodes don't wait the same length of time and immediately cause another collision.

Fortunately, the entire CT scan doesn't need to be re-sent as the information is split into smaller units called *packets*. So only the relevant packet needs to be re-sent, followed by the remaining unsent packets. However if frequent collisions occur, the sending of images can be visibly slowed down.

SHARED SEGMENTS

In figure 1, D (the horizontal line) is the *backbone* of this simple network. D is also a *shared segment*, because many nodes share this "segment" of the network. As this network is so simple, the segment actually comprises the entire backbone, although this isn't normally the case in larger networks, as we shall see.

HUBS

The backbone, D, is normally encased within a piece of network equipment called a *hub*, as below. The term for this internal backbone is a *back plane*.

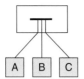

Figure 2

As more nodes are added to this type of single-segment network, and/or as they write more information onto the network, then collisions will occur more frequently. There will be a point where the amount of *network traffic* causes a visible slowing down of the network because of having to wait for a short delay and re-send packets.

A common rule of thumb for Ethernet is that the threshold for an efficient network is 10% of maximum capacity.

Hubs are generally physically separate from each other (e.g. on different floors – one serving C level and one serving D level), and they are joined by the network backbone as below.

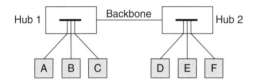

Figure 3

ROUTERS

So if there were capacity problems before the network grew (i.e. with just A, B and C nodes), they will be even worse now with six nodes. However we can add a piece of network equipment called a *router* onto the backbone (R in figure 4). This separates the backbone into two shared segments instead of just one.

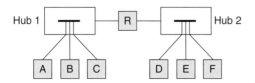

Figure 4

A router looks at the IP addresses of the network traffic, gradually building up a table of where (i.e. in which segment) the various IP addresses live. This is called a *routing table*. Now, when A writes to the network, the router looks at the destination IP address. If the address is in the other segment (i.e. nodes D, E or F) then the router lets the traffic through. If it isn't destined for the other segment, the router won't let it through.

However, there are some drawbacks. Firstly, routers necessitate careful planning of IP addresses in the two segments, so adding a new router into an existing network isn't always easy. Secondly, A's, B's and C's traffic still interfere with each other (as do D's, E's and F's of course). So if PACS network traffic mustn't be slowed down by other traffic, say internet use for example, then all PACS equipment must be on one segment (for example attached to Hub 1), and all other equipment must be on the other segment.

MULTI-SEGMENT HUBS

If all the equipment is physically close together then separating equipment onto separate segments may be achieved using a more advanced hub: a *multi-segment hub*. The two (or more) segments are built into the same piece of equipment. Also, rather than having a separate external router to conditionally join the two segments, the router is often built into the hub too. (R in figure 5).

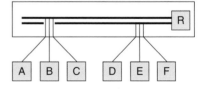

Figure 5

However, in the real world equipment is spread across the campus: the CT scanner and PACS server may be on C level and thus attached to Hub 1 (in figure 4), whilst the main Radiology Department (and associated CR etc) may be on D level, and thus attached to Hub 2. So a significant amount of traffic would still pass through the router, R, reducing the beneficial effect we had hoped for.

SWITCHING

A *switch* addresses the above problem. A "hub" which performs switching is called a *switch*, of which the most common type is the *workgroup switch*. Rather than having a shared segment to which many nodes plug into, each node has its own dedicated segment. In figure 6, when A writes information onto the network destined for C, the switch looks at the destination address and sends it only to C. The traffic doesn't even go onto the backbone, so no router is required.

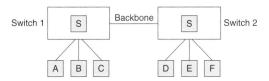

Figure 6

Strictly speaking switches make their decisions on something called a *MAC address*, rather than an IP address, but the concept is still the same. This means that rather than sharing say 100Mb/s between many nodes, node A gets 100Mb/s all to itself, as do all the other nodes. The amount of network bandwidth available to each node has therefore been increased from having just hubs.

Furthermore, even if B starts writing to the network at the same time as A no collision occurs. Collisions are therefore reduced.

MULTI-LAYER SWITCHES

"Layers" in the term *multi-layer switching* refer to the *OSI reference model*. This is a standard way of structuring the many jobs required to achieve networking. Each job is put into a pigeonhole, or *layer*, running from *Application* at layer 7 to *Physical* at layer 1. The job that a MAC address performs lives at layer 2. A MAC address is unique in the whole world, not just within a given network. A MAC address is fixed and is set when any given node is manufactured (or more precisely when the node's network card is manu-

factured). The job that an IP address performs lives at layer 3.

A switch that can look at IP addresses as well as MAC addresses is called either a *layer 3 switch* or a multi-layer switch.

But what's the difference between the two addressing systems? IP addresses aren't just simple addresses like a MAC address is. They are used with something called a *subnet mask*. *Subnetting* is beyond the scope of this book but the effect is that routing an IP address requires some simple calculations. These calculations take a tiny bit longer than switching a MAC address. But when dealing with millions of addresses per second, the time difference is significant. Multi-layer switches therefore calculate a route based on IP address, and make a note of the MAC addresses corresponding to each IP address. Subsequent network traffic is then more efficiently switched based on MAC address. This is called *route once, switch many*.

Finally, there is also some information about the destination contained in the next layer up. Layer 4 includes something called a *port number*. Your web browser reads information from the network only if it is addressed to port number 80 for example. The software running on a PACS workstation will use a different port number. Some switches can also use the port number to decide where to send network traffic. This allows management of network traffic based on the type of traffic, an important step beyond simply managing traffic based on where it has come from or is going to.

We've already seen how segmenting a network helps us to balance the capacity available with the needs of the various types of network users. Multi-layer switching simply gives us a more precise tool for segmenting the network. This is managing the network, i.e. *network management*.

TOKEN RING

Is there a way to improve upon the 10% efficiency threshold of Ethernet? Yes, by controlling when nodes are allowed to write to the network, thus preventing collisions. A *token* travelling around the network, signals that a node may write to the network. Rather than having a backbone, the network is formed into a circle, or *ring*, so that the token continuously cycles around, notifying each node in turn that it may write to the network. This is called a *token ring* network:

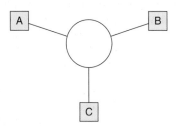

Figure 7

Although a token ring network cannot transfer data as fast as Ethernet (16Mb/s is common), it can function efficiently up to 70% utilisation. This means that the overall network throughput can be higher than with simple Ethernet (70% of 16Mb/s is more than 10% of 100Mb/s).

In practice, the token isn't just a signal but a "container" for the network traffic too. If the token is free, data is written to the network, so the token is in use; no further nodes can write to the network (using that token) until the intended recipient reads the data and marks the token as free again. As more nodes are added, the availability of the token can become a bottleneck. However, a token ring network can have many tokens.

LARGE TOKEN RING NETWORKS

Large token ring networks comprise multiple rings, joined by *bridges*. Bridges are pieces of network equipment similar to routers except they allow all traffic through. They do not examine the destination IP address and then allow or deny the traffic through accordingly; everything goes through.

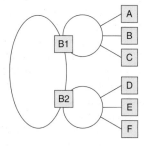

Figure 8

A *campus ring* connects multiple local rings, called *workgroup rings*, together. For example, each floor of a hospital may have its own workgroup ring, all joined to a single campus ring.

FDDI

Frequently the campus ring is a fibre optic cable using a protocol called *FDDI*. For our purposes, FDDI works the same way as token ring. There are some variations in its use of tokens, but these do not help our understanding. FDDI runs at 100Mb/s.

TOKEN RING VERSUS ETHERNET

Token ring had many technical advantages over Ethernet, but the gap has been closed with the advent of switched Ethernet, which removed most of the disadvantages of simple Ethernet. It is also possible to switch token ring networks. But token ring equipment such as switches are all more expensive than their Ethernet counterparts. With the technical issues addressed, Ethernet has established itself as the preferable protocol for most organisations, including hospitals.

ATM

ATM is a switched protocol that is fundamentally different to both Ethernet and token ring. Rather than packets of information gradually finding their way to their intended destination via bridges and routers, etc, an end to end route, or *circuit*, is established when the connection is first made. Contrast this to Ethernet for example where decisions are made about where to route packets when they arrive at any given intermediate piece of network equipment. This processing, as well as other factors, can introduce delays called *latency*. Having a circuit established reduces latency. The packets are called *cells* in ATM jargon, and they are all the same size, which also helps to control latency.

Also ATM does not have shared segments in way that Ethernet and token ring do. The cells from different circuits can be interleaved together (called *multiplexing*), but they do not contend for any shared segment thus risking collisions.

In this way, a guaranteed amount of bandwidth is available. Each node has 155Mb/s all to itself, (155Mb/s is the most common speed for ATM), and ATM can be used close to 100% capacity.

Latency is important for video and voice applications such as videoconferencing because a jittery image is unacceptably distracting. (Do not confuse this type of video with medical cine though, where the whole study is sent to the workstation prior to starting the cine).

ATM VERSUS ETHERNET

The outcome of such a comparison really depends on how the network will be used; each protocol has its own strengths and they should be deployed where those strengths can be capitalised upon.

For example, it isn't usually necessary to have an ATM connection direct to each node (although ATM can using *LAN emulation*). This is because ATM provides more bandwidth than most nodes can use. This includes network intensive nodes such as PACS workstations or spiral CT scanners. So using the cheaper Ethernet protocol to individual nodes, with the switches connected by an ATM backbone is likely to be a "better" solution overall.

But with Ethernet backbones (and even some WAN links) running at 1Gb/s, overall Ethernet may come out ahead of ATM for the backbone, despite ATM's technical superiority.

However, care must be taken that such comparisons are like for like and this may extend beyond simple data. If say, voice is to run over the network too, then ATM may well have many more advantages than Ethernet for data and a separate telephone exchange for voice. When you include a telephone exchange in the comparison, ATM would often be the preferred choice. Because of things like latency, ATM will handle voice much better than Ethernet can – indeed handling voice and video was a key reason for ATM's invention.

So the real answer of which is better is that it depends on your organisation's individual needs.

LAN OR WAN?

So far, we have used examples where all the nodes are in one "local" area. The term "local" is subjective but can be taken to mean anywhere that a node can be connected to the backbone. Generally, this will mean anywhere on a single campus. Such networks are called *local area networks*, or *LANs*.

However, many hospitals are spread across a wider area – usually two (or more) separate campuses. Although each campus has its own LAN, they are linked. The "big picture" view of all the linked campus networks is a *wide area network*, or *WAN*. Often the links themselves are called *WAN links*. Because WAN links cover a much greater distance, often many kilometres, they usually cannot run as fast as a LAN backbone; they have less bandwidth available. WAN links generally have a router at each end. This is to ensure that only traffic that needs to cross the WAN link does so. If only one router were used, then some traffic would cross the WAN link only to be blocked at the other side, thus wasting bandwidth.

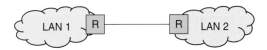

Figure 9

FIREWALLS

A *firewall* is a piece of network equipment that allows or denies traffic to pass through much like a router. However, it is used for security rather than performance reasons. Consider the hospital's WAN to be *trusted*. Any network not owned or controlled by the hospital is not trusted. Two prime examples are the *NHS Net* and the Internet. The NHS Net is a network provided by the Department of Health. Hospitals subscribe to the NHS Net in much the same way that you might subscribe to the internet from home via an *ISP* (*Internet Service Provider*) such as

AOL for example. All traffic going to or coming from a network that is not trusted must pass through the firewall first.

Take the example of a PC owned by another hospital, for example a neurological specialist centre, to which you wish to allow access from your network. Rules would be written telling the firewall to allow your PACS server to access this PC. The firewall identifies traffic as coming from your PACS server by its IP address, and identifies the PC by the destination IP address. So the firewall allows the traffic to pass through. You can write rules so that the firewall allows traffic in one direction only (i.e. allowing your PACS server to "push" images but preventing the PC from "pulling" them), or so that it allows traffic in both directions. However no other PCs (nor any other nodes) at that neurological specialist centre are allowed access to the PACS server; they are blocked by the firewall.

Additionally, the rules can include a port number (see Multi-layer switches), which define the type of traffic. Thus, you may be able to access the Internet from your hospital PC because the firewall allows traffic through only if the traffic is destined for port 80. However someone trying to *hack* into your PC via the Internet would be thwarted because the firewall would block all attempts to access other ports, for example the ones relevant to transferring files, or to access the PACS. The solution isn't perfect of course – you can still download virus-infected files from the Internet (i.e. via port 80) – but a firewall is an essential and significant part of any *network security policy*.

Finally, a firewall can perform *IP address mapping* or *IP address translation*. Recall that an IP address can be duplicated in another network so long as the two networks are never connected. Well, a node on the Internet could well be using the same IP address as is currently allocated to your PC at work. So the firewall maps your existing IP address to another one – one from a small range of IP addresses allocated to the hospital that are guaranteed to be unique on the Internet. These addresses are called *public* IP addresses, and the hospital will no doubt have many more nodes than it has public IP addresses. So the firewall maps the *private* IP addresses to public ones and vice versa before letting the traffic pass through.

REAL WORLD NETWORKS

Although older PACS implementations are running on older, slower networks, the progression of bandwidth requirements from devices such as spiral CT scanners has increased the "minimum specification" for PACS networks. This trend can be expected to continue with for example mammography and non-radiographic imaging such as pathology and medical photography.

It is generally accepted that modalities and PACS workstations should be supplied with 100Mb/s. These should then be linked to a "significant" backbone, such as ATM or 1Gb/s Ethernet. In any case, the network must be switched. WAN links vary depending on application. For example, a remote site doing only a few ultrasound studies may cope quite adequately with a *dial-up connection* (i.e. up to 128Kb/s). A higher throughput of studies and/or more demanding imaging such as CR would probably necessitate a 100Mb/s WAN link. However, a large hospital spread evenly between two campuses may require an ATM or 1Gb/s Ethernet WAN link between the campuses.

Finally, we must address the issue of separate networks. Traffic congestion on the network caused by one application can affect the performance of an unrelated application (e.g. PACS), sharing the same network. PACS vendors understandably therefore wish to keep PACS separate by having a separate physical network – separate cabling, separate switches and separate workstations.

However I believe it is in hospitals' immediate and long-term interests *not* to have a separate network. Why shouldn't a clinician have only one PC in their office running both PACS and HIS? Why have two switches side by side, neither using more than a few percent of their capacity? Having a separate network hinders work practices, thus limiting benefits that may otherwise be gained. It also wastes space and costs more.

Of course, the vendors concerns *must* be addressed. In the end, they are your concerns too. And they can be addressed by *logically* separating the PACS network. Modern network equipment can do this, guaranteeing bandwidth for PACS, if necessary at the expense of other applications. Such advanced networking is beyond the scope of this book, but for the interested reader, logical separation revolves around *VLANs* and *quality of service*, or *QoS*.

INTERFACING

We have so far discussed to some degree the five major component systems that comprise a PACS:

- HIS
- RIS
- PACS
- Modalities
- Interfaces, including networks

We can now follow their functions through to arrive at an overall PACS system meaningful to the needs of a hospital.

Note that people will call the overall system "PACS", and care must be taken to avoid confusing this meaning with that of the PACS server & software. In this book where a distinction is required we will use the phrase "PACS subsystem" to refer to the PACS server, software and workstations.

We can think of interfacing two systems together in terms of them having a "conversation". If we were to ask the HIS and RIS suppliers to write a direct interface to each other, then the resultant "conversation" between the two systems would be a "private conversation". Even if the subject of the conversation would be of interest to PACS, for example patient demographics, PACS would still not be able to "listen in" on those parts of the conversation that it was interested in. This type of interface is called a proprietary interface. A proprietary interface between HIS and RIS would necessitate a completely new and separate interface between HIS and PACS for them to communicate.

INTERFACE ENGINES

Introducing the concept of an interface engine saves such duplication. Patient demographics are already being sent by HIS to RIS. If these are sent via an interface engine (i/f) then when PACS is installed, it can "tap into" the HIS/RIS conversation as per the diagram. This reduces duplication of effort, as there is only one outgoing HIS interface.

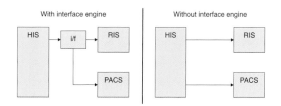

Figure 10

TRANSLATIONS

Another job that the interface engine has to perform is "translations". For example the gender field of HIS may be male, female, indeterminate or unknown, represented by 'M', 'F', 'I' and ' ' (space) respectively. RIS and PACS may only store male, female, and unknown, although these could well be represented by 'M', 'F' and 'U'. The interface engine would therefore perform the following translations, also called "mappings":

- 'M' -> 'M'
- 'F' -> 'F'
- 'I' -> 'U'
- ' ' -> 'U'

DATA FORMATS

Another type of translation is of formats. For example if the HIS is reasonably old, it might only send out data in proprietary format rather than a standard format such as "HL7". The engine would then translate the proprietary data format from HIS to HL7 before forwarding on to other hospital systems. Another simple example is between comma separated and fixed length formats – you can experiment with these yourself by importing text files into any popular spreadsheet. Figure 11 shows the same data (surname, forename, sex and date of birth) in both formats.

| Oakley, Jason, M, 19570215 | Oakley   Jason   M19570215 |
| Smith, Annabelle, F, 19790927 | Smith   Annabelle   F19790927 |

Figure 11

You can see that in the left-hand column the commas separate each part of the data or "field". The comma is called the "field separator" or "field delimiter". Each field is therefore variable length. The right-hand column is fixed length format. Each field starts at the same column position, so fields that are too short are padded with spaces to achieve the same fixed width. Conversely, if a forename were longer than 9 characters, then the forename would have to be truncated.

Because the interface engine will need to talk to systems from multiple suppliers, it will most likely be "open", meaning non-proprietary. For example to describe what the next chunk of data will be, a supplier could unilaterally decide on the descriptor "DEMO" to describe demographic data. Although sensible it would be better to use a descriptor that everyone else uses such as one from an accepted standard. HL7 is a prime example of such a standard. A system which adheres to accepted standards can be described as an "open system". HL7's descriptor for patient basic details including demographics is "PID". HL7 also has variable length fields, analogous to the comma-separated example above, although it uses a vertical bar or "pipe" symbol (|) as a field delimiter and even has sub-fields, which are delimited by a caret (^).

SELECTIVITY

Another job that the interface engine performs is that of selectivity. In our conversation analogy PACS is only interested in demographics. However, although both PACS and RIS are interested in demographics, RIS is only interested in demographics for patients that RIS is going to "see", i.e. those patients that will visit the Radiology department. PACS however is interested in all patients because while the patient is in the hospital potentially any speciality might want to review previous images. So the interface engine receives demographics for all patients and forwards all of them to PACS. But it only forwards demographics to RIS if the patient location is set to "Radiology".

You can now see the way systems are interfaced together to reflect the workings of the hospital. Defining the interfaces therefore is not solely the task of technical personnel as they will not be familiar with the clinical workflow that the data represents; it requires both clinicians and technical staff working together. Furthermore, because work practices are significantly different between plain film and PACS it makes it even harder to define interfaces.

PACS BROKER

The above jobs that an interface engine performs are as applicable to banking or engineering applications as they are to healthcare. However there are other tasks, specific to PACS, for which a specialised type of interface engine is required − a PACS Broker, or simply broker. A PACS Broker translates certain non-image components of DICOM to HL7 and vice-versa.

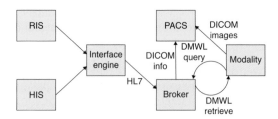

Figure 12

WORK LISTS

The list of patients that are scheduled to be imaged at a given modality is called a work list. The DICOM term for this is DICOM Modality Work List, or DMWL. In figure 12 RIS sends a list of patients that are to be imaged to the interface engine, which then forwards it to the PACS Broker, which stores the list. At regular intervals (e.g. every 1 or 5 minutes), the modalities *query/retrieve* from the broker their latest work list of patients that are to be imaged *that day*. This act of regularly getting the latest list is called polling the broker.

At the modality itself, the radiographer doesn't need to type the patient details again (e.g. name, date of birth, etc) but merely associates the images with the existing patient details from the work list.

When the radiographer indicates on RIS that the procedure has been ended, (see Tracking Functions in Chapter 6 – RIS) this is sent across the interface to the PACS Broker. The PACS Broker can then remove the patient from the modality's work list, thus keeping the work list to a manageable size.

BENEFITS OF INTERFACING

This tight integration allows PACS to realise one of its major benefits – no lost or mis-filed "films". Because every image is associated with accurate patient details, subsequent searches will find both the correct patient and every image in PACS of that patient. Note that other mechanisms, for example bar coding of image plates in CR, do not prevent associating an image with a completely different patient.

Work lists, and the reduced inputting and errors that they confer, also contribute to higher patient throughput in a PACS environment. This is also a more tangible benefit than less lost films – good for those staff justifying a PACS business case – because to measure a reduction in lost films you need to know how many are being lost pre-PACS. And to accurately count how many, you would need to find all the lost films first!

DATA QUALITY

Work lists aren't just a nicety to save the radiographer some typing. They also improve data quality. The unfortunate case of a death from meningococcal meningitis where poor data quality was a contributing factor (albeit out of several hospital errors) highlighted its importance and in fact helped get the message across to users. This applied and applies to everyone who enters data, directly or indirectly, from senior clinicians to clerks.

The IT aspect of the case was that the patient was duplicated on the system several times, but with mis-spelt surnames and an incorrect date of birth, thus preventing the ward from finding Pathology results for the patient.

BEYOND THE RADIOLOGY DEPARTMENT

Even when measured against all the above benefits, the high cost, effort and expertise required for interfacing may still not immediately add up. However, remember that we are building *infrastructure*. And this interfacing forms part of the hospital's infrastructure, not just that of the PACS or the Radiology Department. Indeed almost all hospitals will already have an interface engine of some description, for example for HIS to Pathology interfacing. Interfacing to HIS is also a pre-requisite for deploying PACS beyond the Radiology Department.

To understand why, first recall from Chapter 3 – Equipment, that hard disk storage is fast but can hold relatively few images. Archive storage (i.e. tape or CD-ROM or DVD jukeboxes) can hold vast numbers of images but is relatively slow.

But having an interface from HIS to PACS means that images can be pre-fetched from archive to the much faster hard disk in the evening prior to their use – for example for an orthopaedic outpatient appointment the next day. HIS holds all the hospital's outpatient clinic lists, and can send details of the next day's patients to PACS each night (via the interface engine of course). This means that the orthopaedic surgeon in clinic has instant access to all the patient's previous images – no waiting for retrieval from archive.

The trigger to pre-fetch must in this case come from HIS not RIS, as follow-up patients especially may not need any further imaging. Also for those PACS that employ auto-forwarding, the HIS outpatient booking will have details of the clinic, room and consultant which will be used by the PACS sub-system to determine which workstation(s) to auto-forward images to.

What if the patient isn't on PACS, for example if they've never been imaged? The PACS sub-system simply discards the trigger to pre-fetch. The interface engine cannot be selective here without holding a duplicate of the PACS subsystem's patient index, which would be inefficient. The interface engine is still being selective, albeit at a coarser level, by not forwarding irrelevant outpatient clinic details, for example for a dermatology clinic.

Similarly, accident & emergency and intensive

care admissions can be made to trigger pre-fetching. Even though in these specialities the number of cases where previous images are used for management of the patient is low, the images are at least there for the times when they are useful. This benefit is simply not practical in a non-interfaced PACS environment. It is capitalising on the interface infrastructure.

In any case PACS still needs to know when a patient is admitted or discharged from intensive care. A protracted episode in intensive care can easily have images taken at the start of the episode beyond the time where they would usually "fall off" hard disk storage. By knowing that the patient hasn't been discharged from intensive care yet, the PACS can retain those images on fast hard disk storage for immediate access.

So interfacing lets PACS realise more of its benefits; with RIS, it improves data quality and throughput. With HIS, it enables deployment beyond the Radiology Department. But what about beyond the hospital itself – tertiary referrals and GP referrals for example?

WEB SERVER

A PACS web server allows staff to view PACS images using a web browser. You can think of the web browser as another type of PACS workstation, except web browsers are easier and cheaper to deploy throughout the hospital and beyond. The trade-off is that the web browser will have less PACS functions than dedicated viewing software provided by your PACS supplier.

The PACS web server itself is just another integral component of the PACS sub-system designed to handle the connections from the web browsers. However, they generally work by taking a subset of images that are on the main PACS server, having converted them into a format suitable web browsers. This format can be lossy compressed if it suits working practices (for example for General Practitioners who use the report more than the image). The subset may be defined by information interfaced from RIS, for example certain modalities, or from HIS, for example referring GP, or a combination of both.

TERTIARY REFERRALS

In the scenarios so far, the PACS sub-system has used information interfaced from other hospital systems to minimise (or even remove) manual intervention to make images readily available to clinicians at the point of use. PACS has removed the manual process of "pulling notes."

However from the HIS' point of view, an outgoing tertiary referral – where the patient is sent to a local specialist centre – is no different to a simple discharge. Although the HIS will have a "Discharged To" field, this will only hold a value such as "Tertiary Referral Centre". How would PACS know that the referral was to say a neurological specialist centre, in which case CT head scans would be relevant to send, but CR chest images irrelevant? Or indeed the referral could be to an intensive care unit, where CR chest images might be key to management of the patient?

Unfortunately, the solution here is manual intervention. Any of the possible local destinations (the neurological specialist centre and the intensive care unit in our example) need to have a *DICOM workstation*. I am using the term DICOM workstation because the centre does not need to have a PACS system. A DICOM workstation can be as simple as one PC with *DICOM viewing software* to display the images. Someone from your hospital must manually select the appropriate images from your PACS and send them to the appropriate destination. Defining the "appropriate destination," i.e. a *DICOM destination* is a technical task; defining who that "someone" may be is a work-practice issue.

DEFINING DICOM DESTINATIONS

A *DICOM destination* has an *Application Entity Title* (*AE Title*) and *port number*, which can be thought of as its DICOM address, and an *IP address*, which is its network address. The tertiary hospital provides these details. They can find the AE Title and port number in the "set up," "settings" or configuration details of the DICOM viewing software. They can also find the IP address in the corresponding part of the *operating system* software (e.g. Windows or Unix).

IP addresses are a bit "them and us" so the tertiary hospital's IP address must be *translated* into an IP address suitable for your hospital. This is done by the *firewall*. (See the Firewall section for an explanation why).

You then enter them (the AE Title, port number and *your* version of their IP address) into your PACS to define the new destination that you are creating.

These are the minimum requirements to be able to forward images on from the PACS, in this case to a tertiary referral centre. Additionally, for security the DICOM viewing software might only accept images from specific sources. So the tertiary hospital may also need to enter details of your PACS into the tertiary hospital's DICOM viewing software.

In practice, the set up and testing DICOM destinations is error-prone and errors are frustratingly difficult to trace. This is partly because of how firewalls work. When they block traffic they do so silently – they don't respond with an error message saying, "This traffic has been blocked because of x". Also setting up a DICOM destination frequently involves six separate groups staff – PACS staff from each hospital (often from the Radiology Department), networking/firewall staff from each hospital, *field engineers* from the PACS supplier and finally field engineers for the DICOM workstation.

DISTRIBUTION SERVER

PACS uses a method called *DICOM store* to store images on the tertiary hospital's DICOM workstation, just as modalities use DICOM store when they send images to PACS. However, many PACS suppliers view the PACS server as "incoming" only, so they design it to only accept DICOM store requests (e.g. from modalities), but not to issue them (e.g. to tertiary hospitals' workstations). So the job of sending images from PACS is often performed by another component of the PACS sub-system called a *distribution server*. The PACS server copies images directly onto the distribution server in the same way that it copies images to the archive.

The distribution server can also perform *encryption* and compression before forwarding the images. Encryption means scrambling the images so that only the intended recipient can unscramble them (and thereby view them). The distribution server can also vary the degree of encryption according to where the images are going. For example using strong encryption if the images are to go across the Internet, and no encryption (or a weak but fast encryption) for images going over a more trusted network such as the NHS Net.

The distribution server can also make similar decisions about compression (Chapter Eight – Image Manipulation). For example, if the image's destination were a tertiary referral centre, where image quality is paramount, then the distribution server would apply lossless compression. However, because General Practitioners rely on the radiologist's report, image quality is less important, so the distribution server would decide that lossy compression is more appropriate (whether GPs access images through the distribution server or the web server depends on the PACS system purchased).

Of course, the hospital must define the distribution server's rules to apply a given type of encryption and compression according to image destination.

ORDER COMMUNICATIONS

The final interfacing subject returns to within the hospital. *Order communications* or *OC* describes a system that takes clinical orders or requests, rather than using paper request cards.

OC is sometimes a module within HIS, and sometimes a separate system. Radiology OC is interfaced to the RIS. Although completely separate from PACS, it still benefits PACS users.

If PACS workstations can also run RIS (or if OC details are interfaced to PACS), then the radiologist can report from any PACS workstation. They are not tied to where the physical list of paper request cards are kept, and can therefore report from their offices, a separate building, or a remote hospital site. Rather than spending additional time travelling, they can report from wherever is most efficient.

This is an example of the pervasive benefits of interfacing. Its effects ripple beyond staff grade and departmental boundaries, making work-practices more efficient and adding new benefits long after initial implementation, thus progressively reinforcing the thought, "How did we ever cope without PACS."

6: RADIOLOGY INFORMATION SYSTEMS

Jason Oakley

INTRODUCTION

Previous chapters have dealt firstly with standards that allow computers to interface, namely DICOM and HL7 and then with basic network design and set up. Together, these standards and the technologies that they support should allow all systems within a healthcare environment to communicate seamlessly. The reality can be very different from this.

This chapter will look at the functions one can expect to be part of a radiology information system (RIS) and why they are important in the running of an imaging service. The chapter will also explore some of the difficulties that come with any RIS and how they can be overcome. Chapter 11 will deal with the radiographers and radiologists experiences of actually working with such systems, and this chapter will dwell only briefly on the potential frustrations of users, concentrating more on the technical issues that surround such information databases.

The chapter that follows this one, Picture Archiving and Communications Systems, will examine how all of the systems related to imaging can fit together in the wider hospital network.

An understanding of RIS is important for a number of reasons;

- Realising the importance of RIS encourages good data entry
- RIS is not that dissimilar from other departmental systems so the principles are transferable
- Knowing how the RIS works enables the user to move faster around the sub pages when locating or inputting data
- Knowing what the RIS can do means that you will get the most from the system

HISTORY IN PERSPECTIVE

It is not that long ago that all information in imaging departments was recorded manually onto paper (and this is still the case in some smaller clinics). This often took the form of day sheets, which recorded the date, time, patient details, examination and appointment time. A patient would have a paper x-ray record that listed these details and within which the typed reports from multiple examinations could be stored. A carbon copy of any typed report would be sent to the referring clinician whose responsibility it was to place the report in the appropriate section of the notes.

This system, which worked perfectly well for years had several distinct disadvantages;

- Legibility of data recorded (both hand written and carbon copies)
- All records had to be physically retrieved by hand
- No single point for retrieval of information
- Easy for records to become lost
- Easy for duplicate examinations to be carried out
- All data has to be re-recorded at every point of patient contact

Another previously unrealised disadvantage was the lack of utility that this data offered by virtue of being stored on paper. As an example let us consider a researcher hoping to establish a link between patient's age and primary lung cancers. All of the information required has been recorded and we will assume that no records are lost and that all information has been recorded legibly.

The only way to perform this search would be to first go through every single day sheet for a period of time looking for patients who attended for chest x-rays. After recording each of the patient details each of the patients' reports could be pulled and read, looking for reports that indicated a primary lung neoplasm. This would mean wading through thousands of irrelevant reports in order to identify the very small study group.

Large-scale studies have previously required extensive resources in order to acquire such data. Now the computer allows a far faster and systematic search of patient information. If we use the same example the researcher could easily ask (with the appropriate security access) for all chest x-ray reports to be listed containing certain keywords. Such as neoplasm, cancer, mass etc which would massively reduce the number of reports needing to be read through to obtain the required data. The computer would also perform the search and collate the information far faster and more efficiently than any human could hope too.

But a radiology information system is capable of far more than this as will become clear later in this chapter.

Basic RIS have been around for some time, allowing the input of patient details, appointments, etc but these systems, whilst performing an invaluable service at the time, have now left many departments with a potentially expensive problem. Many of the older systems utilised stand-alone terminals that could only be used for the RIS and were linked simply to a local network. Because each of the terminals only had to communicate with the RIS computer it didn't matter if the language used was proprietary, i.e. specific to that manufacturer.

Now the personal computer (PC) is replacing these terminal based systems allowing multiple applications to be run alongside the RIS. This means that each point of interface (the PC) has more than one use. The same computer can now be used to access the Internet, review images on the PACS, retrieve e-mails etc.

The problem with the proprietary systems was that a wealth of data had been built up on RIS, i.e. patient information, reports etc, but it was all in a supplier specific language. The choices are to:

- Pay for the information to be translated onto the new system, which may be expensive and also very time consuming
- Run the new and old systems side by side for a period of years (very unsatisfactory working environment)
- Discard old information (unworkable)

However, providing such systems have been put in place and that transfer of information to the new RIS is possible, the modern system can start to provide information as soon as it is running.

The changeover from an existing system must be planned well, as any unforeseen downtime can have a major impact on the efficiency of the imaging department.

RIS AND HIS

At this present time RIS should be considered a stand-alone system that manages information generated in the imaging department. It is specific for that purpose and is not a transferable system that could be used in the histo-pathology department. In the same way that other departments systems would be quite unsuitable for use in an imaging department.

The Hospital Information System (HIS) should be considered as the central repository of patient information (often called the Patient Master Index, or PMI). This will include patient name, date of birth, address, patient episodes etc, for a range of sub-systems in place around the hospital, as well as those solely entered on the HIS. Figure 1 shows the HIS as the hub of a wider network of patient information.

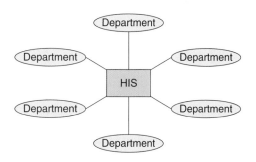

Figure 1 – Centralised HIS

The first thing that is assumed is that the HIS and the RIS can in fact interface. If this is not possible then either the HIS or the RIS have been inappropriately purchased. There is little point, within the modern NHS, in having systems that cannot communicate as this will not move a hospital towards achieving a totally electronic patient record (EPR).

Having said that the systems **must** interface, it is not always the case that systems can be simply connected together and then expected to communicate meaningfully with each other. It is more often the case that the two systems will require some form of interface engine to correct the differences between the data streams. This can even be the case in systems which both claim to be HL7 compliant.

The HIS is normally considered the reference point for all information and it is therefore the most important database to be accurate and up to date. For this reason only certain individuals with have access to inputting data into the HIS to ensure minimum errors. This means that as far as the RIS is concerned the HIS is a source of information as well as a receiver of information.

It is often assumed that RIS and HIS are inter-active, with the RIS updating the HIS and vice versa (figure 2).

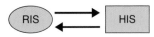

Figure 2 – HIS/RIS interface

However figure 3 is actually far more accurate.

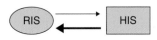

Figure 3 – Actual HIS/RIS interface

Because of worries of incorrect patient data entry, or potential mis-use of patient data the RIS actually only draws information from the HIS. This should reduce errors in data entry in radiol-ogy but does mean that if a patient advises the radiographer that their details are incorrect they are unable to correct them on the HIS. They could correct them on the RIS, and it is often believed that this will then update the HIS, but this is rarely the case.

It is not uncommon for a single individual to be trained to use a separate terminal to correct HIS data or, as was the authors experience, to have to telephone a central number to advise a HIS operator of any changes that were required.

There is, however, now a growing acceptance that, as more of the staff within a hospital become more familiar with computers, there should be more updating of the HIS by remote systems, such as RIS. It is often the health care worker dealing with a patient, face to face, who has the most up to date information regarding that patient. Patients' names and date of birth (DOB) are often checked as part of a standard identification protocol within a department and it is here that spelling mistakes, or inaccurate DOB's are spotted. It must be considered best practise for the person who is informed of the error (or who picks it up by way of a standard "who are you" identification protocol) to be able to correct the data there and then on their departmental system. If this is not done then the incorrect details are continued until corrected at a later stage, again by someone remote from the patient.

This does introduce some new issues, as it would mean that a whole new level of staff would need to have access to a far wider level of information, again opening up security issues. The main worry would still be that information could be altered incorrectly meaning that the patient information is potentially lost.

This may seem unrealistic, but if a patient's data was being corrected from *Oakley, John* to *Oakley, Jason* but during inputting the operator typed *9Oakley, Jason* and did not notice their mistake, then retrieving that data via the name would be almost impossible. Advanced searches on more modern RIS can help in the location of this type of misnamed file, but such searches can be laborious.

If the network connection to the HIS goes down, or if the HIS itself has any downtime this will have an immediate effect on the RIS. When a patient's information is requested, the RIS will be unable to find the data and will assume that the patient is new. This may require the user to input all available patient data into the RIS in order to proceed with the examination. A deci-sion (or better yet a departmental protocol designed to cope with this eventuality) must be made to cover what needs to be done. Does the user input all available patient data as a new patient in order to continue with the examina-tion, or store the details elsewhere until the HIS becomes active again and then use the HIS details as normal? If the RIS is capable of updat-ing HIS then inputting minimum patient details would allow the patient to be recorded onto the system and any updating done later. If the deci-sion is to wait until HIS is back running and then add the patient this can result in the same exam-ination being performed twice (unnecessarily) as the HIS could be several days out of date.

RIS AND PACS

It is also worth mentioning that a RIS is not the same as a PACS. A RIS can be thought of as a text based information system, whilst a PACS is very much an image based information system. This does not mean that a RIS could not be part of a PACS. It very much depends on the set up of the individual systems. The RIS should always be considered as dealing with the textual information generated by the imaging department, including the location of film packets, but it does not deal with the actual images themselves.

The PACS is a way of managing the images themselves, but the information regarding the patient within the image will have come from the RIS that will in turn have got the information from the HIS. Figure 4 explains this process.

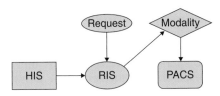

Figure 4 – RIS and PACS connection

In this flowchart we can see that a request is presented and the patient's information drawn from the RIS. This will create a work list for the modality, which will be sent to the modality on the day of the examination (or upon request from the modality). The modality will use this information to add patient details to the images, and then add modality specific information to the file. This file would normally be created to the DICOM standard. These images will then subsequently be sent to the PACS. It may of course be the PACS that creates the work list so the connection with the modality for the RIS may be through the PACS itself.

Connectivity is again an important issue. Ideally there should be seamless integration between all systems and this may be achieved using an interface engine. However, it is still possible for the information to be transferred incorrectly or unreliably because one system can misinterpret characters used by the other system. This can introduce the step of re-inputting information or printing out barcodes that can then be used to input the data onto the new system. Whatever the solution might be to this it is better if the connectivity problems are

solved initially and secondary fixes are avoided wherever possible.

It will be mentioned in other chapters but it is worth reiterating that users of computer systems expect far more from them than they would from a paper system. They know that interfacing can be done and will see it as a failure of the management or the vendors if this integration is not done seamlessly and fully.

It is very likely that the newer RIS in the market place will be HL7 systems and this will mean that there is a good chance of a good interface being achieved, even if it has to be through an interface engine. Older systems operate on standards other than HL7 and interfacing in the long term is probably unrealistic.

RIS AND ORDER COMMUNICATIONS

Order Communications (OC or OCM) is a step towards completely removing all paper systems from the health care environment. OC allows a doctor or other health care professional on the ward to order any test that they need utilising a terminal rather than filling out a paper form. The referrer can select the patient they need the test on, add an appropriate reason to the electronic request and then electronically sign it using a unique identifying code.

This request is then sent to the network that routes it to the RIS (or other hospital system, as appropriate), where the request is either looked at by a human or automatically vetted by the system. An appointment is then allocated and the porters ordered using the same OC message triggers. The advantages are an increase in the speed with which requests are sent and received, and the removal of lost forms from the potential list of delays to a patient's diagnosis and treatment.

A disadvantage might be that the automated ordering means that the referrer could have a drop down list of reasons for each x-ray request, and if their reason does not fit within this strict criterion, they will pick the nearest thing. Another problem is that electronic signatures or personal identification numbers (PINs) are often passed onto other people without question or thought to the consequences. Most people are happy for other members of their family to know their PIN for their cash card, and so are quite happy for others to input data under their log in on a computer.

Would they be as happy to see someone signing their name on a sheet of paper? It is this change of mind set that is required if the electronic patient record is to become as reliable as its paper counterpart.

Interfacing with the OC has the same issues of ensuring that the systems communicate with as little trouble as possible. OC is at this time relatively untested and issues will continue to arise as its implementation becomes more widespread.

BASIC RIS SET-UP

Figure 5 shows the RIS in the context of the network and other departments.

In this example a number of sites are connected to the main RIS network via servers and routers. The RIS itself is responsible for requesting and drawing information from the HIS via the network. The PACS is able to request details from both the RIS and the HIS using the network. The other departmental systems are able to use the network to communicate with the HIS.

The potential also exists for their terminals to access the RIS and the PACS, to varying levels. The variety of set ups is almost unlimited, but will normally be governed by existing systems and network limitations and cost.

FUNCTIONS WITHIN RIS

The function of a RIS is to allow patient information to be inputted, stored and retrieved in as simple a manner as possible. The RIS must then manage the data in such a way as to glean as much benefit from it as possible.

RIS has functions that are designed to mimic previous paper systems plus a number of other functions that increase the ease with which information can be extracted. Every manufacturer's system will have the basic capabilities but the advanced functions will vary from manufacturer to manufacturer. The names and terms used will also be different but it is normally apparent what function they perform.

Log On
A RIS must require every user to log on in order to access any function, and ideally no other user should use a terminal that is logged onto someone else's account. The reason for this is so that there is a traceable train of events. Figure 6 emphasises this point.

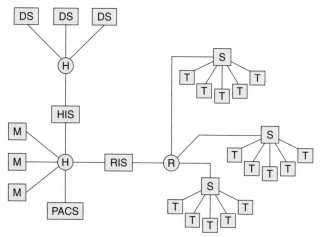

KEY

DS – Departmental Systems
H – Hub or switch
HIS – Hospital Information System
M – Modalities
PACS – Picture Archiving and Communications System
R – Router
RIS – Radiology Information System
S – Server
T – Terminals

Figure 5 – RIS in the wider context

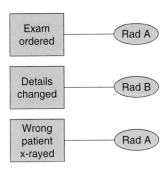

Figure 6 – Traceable chain of events

In this example it would be relatively easy to go back and work out that the patient details had been altered and this resulted in the wrong patient being x-rayed. But this information is of little use without knowing who performed which part of the procedure. This is not necessarily for proving guilt, but more for ensuring that the mistake that was made last time is not made again. It may be that working practices or inappropriate training are the main culprits.

In the same way it would be of little use if Rad A left the terminal logged on and during that time Rad B came along and altered the patient demographics. After the error has occurred the computer would show that all events that occurred to the patient's data were performed by Rad A. It is their electronic signature on the computer, and therefore their responsibility. However inconvenient it may be it is very important to log on when you are using a system and to ensure that you log off when finished. An interesting point of discussion here is whose responsibility is it to log on/off. There is as much a responsibility for the person who goes to use a terminal already logged on to log it off and then log on as themselves, as it is for the user leaving the terminal to remember to log off. If you were to enter an examination room and find a patient already on the table – would you take over the examination? No – you would either leave the room to find somewhere else to do your own examination or track down the person who left the patient on the table to see if it is appropriate for you to remove them from the room. The same should be said for the computer systems – it may be left logged on for a valid reason (user

called away to an emergency – or a search is being run that is taking an extended length of time. If the search is interrupted this will tie the terminal up for the same amount of time again.

Administrative Functions

These are simple functions that allow information to be looked at. For example if a patient was presenting for a certain examination and asked which doctor the results would be going back to the name of the GP could be found here, along with other basic information. This information is drawn from the HIS and is normally not alterable. If the information is altered it will often only update the RIS and not the HIS. Being able to alter the information is often a reserved function, requiring a higher level of access.

Ordering

Ordering is either requesting an examination to be done as soon as is possible or alternatively ordering it for a specific appointment time. All that is normally required to pull up the patient's information is the name and date of birth or a unique identifier. This will then draw all of the patient's information from the HIS.

Most systems will then advise the user of any suspected duplicate patients, similar either by name or number. Some systems take these suspected duplicates a little further and will have a spread of birth dates that will count towards warning the user of a similar patient. For example Jason Oakley 11.04.1970 may be counted in a suspected duplicate for John Oakley 11.05.1973, even though to the human eye these two patients are obviously different.

Once this screen is confirmed the operator then inputs the examination required. This is normally done using either a drop down screen that lists all examinations, or via a list of codes such as RFT for right foot. The RIS automatically puts in all other relevant pieces of the patients data.

Once all of the details of the examination have been confirmed and an event has been triggered on the RIS, the patient can then proceed to have their examination. If an order has not been made then the patient should not be able to have the procedure started.

At this point it is perhaps appropriate to raise the question of what to do with unidentified patients (the unknowns in A&E etc.) As the whole point of having all these systems is to integrate everything into the EPR, if you allow the unknowns to be imaged without inputting the details onto your RIS you can not update the EPR for that patient once their details become known. The department also loses the physical proof of examination, so it will appear they do less work than is actually done. Obviously once you agree how to deal with the unknown or uncommunicative patients you need to think about how you manage the merging of these details onto RIS.

Order Modification

Order modification allows an order that has been previously input to be changed. It could be something as simple as a change from left to right or it could be adding together a number of other examinations. The ability to add examinations together is very important, as it will prevent a patient having to have multiple visits to the department for procedures that could have been done together.

Order Cancellation

It is not uncommon for procedures to be cancelled in light of changes in the patient's condition or management. It is necessary to then be able to cancel an examination, but the information regarding the examination is still kept. This is made useful by the person cancelling having to input the reason why the examination is being cancelled, such as at Doctor's request. This data can then be used if there is a query over who cancelled the request, or why it was not done.

Scheduling

Scheduling can incorporate ordering, but it instead deals with the allocation of specific time slots for appointments. Functions within this allow resources within the department to be viewed. These resources can be rooms, allowing rooms to be blocked out during holiday periods or staff shortages or extra slots can be added for extra sessions. Sometimes it is not the room that is the problem, it is the operator availability that is important (such as a specific radiologist for a particular examination).

Scheduling can be set up so that as soon as an appointment is made the correct patient information letter is sent along with advice on the procedure itself.

Scheduling can also be used to allocate staff to rooms once the usage has been determined. All of these functions should make for a more efficient department.

Scheduling also has a major benefit when multiple healthcare providers are linked together using the same RIS (Figure 7).

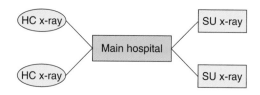

Figure 7 – Remote scheduling

In this set up there are two health centre (HC) x-ray departments and two satellite unit (SU) x-ray departments. These have full access to the RIS and patients referred for simple procedures to any department can be offered the first appointment in the hospital of their choice. It may be that the HCs have a short wait for routine x-rays, and if the patient is willing to travel then they can have their x-ray done sooner. This makes far better use of the resources available in the region as a whole as well as in the immediate location.

Tracking Functions

Tracking is the inputting of data as a patient goes through an examination or procedure. When the patient's examination is first ordered the patient is effectively waiting for the time of the examination to come. When the patient actually arrives this should be input into the system. The time the patient is actually waiting for the procedure to start is now being recorded.

Once the patient comes into the x-ray room the procedure has begun and the examination is then undertaken. When the examination is over and the patient has left the procedure can be ended, thus recording the total time of the episode.

The ending of the procedure is very important as several pieces of information are recorded here;

- Radiographer/radiologist
- Room examination performed in

- Number and size of films used
- Number of repeats taken
- Radiographer/radiologists comments
- Exposure details

If incorrect details are recorded then the data is practically useless, limiting the value of the RIS to the department.

Tracking should be undertaken in real time in order that the information recorded is as accurate as possible, but this is often not possible in the clinical situation. A facility normally exists to belatedly track patients or to end the examination without using times, but still record the number of films etc that were used. For every bit of information missed, the utility of the RIS is reduced.

Equally important is the ability to find out which patients have not been tracked and to check that the examinations have been done and attribute the episode to a radiographer or radiologist.

Film File

This is used when the RIS is being used in conjunction with a conventional film/screen combination and a film library requires management for the vast array of film packets stored within it. It effectively replaces the old card system with an electronic database of who has films and for how long. When a film is requested the person taking it is recorded and a time scale selected for its return. The system can again be automated so that when a film has been out for a certain amount of time a letter is sent requesting its return. This type of automatic tracking of films can be very useful to the department as a whole because the RIS will show at a glance who was last responsible for the film packet. Thus if a repeat request is made from a clinician because of lost films, the culprit can be traced and hopefully the films can be retrieved without further exposure of the patient. This is one of the prime examples of the GIGO syndrome (Garbage In, Garbage Out) where users often find the task of inputting the data tedious and/or time consuming (and so do not do it). Would this attitude change if they had an overall concept of the reason and benefits for the action?

The use of a database allows other users to determine where the film is if they wish to look at it, and how long that other person has had the films.

Clinics that require large quantities of films can have access to a limited part of the RIS that allows them to request x-rays direct from their clinic lists. These are listed as work lists for the library staff in advance of the clinic and they pull the films and send them to the clinic. The RIS knows where the films have gone, and will allocate a certain time limit for their return. In an ideal world where HIS and RIS integration are seamless, HIS would supply clinic lists to RIS automatically at a predetermined time prior to the actual date of clinic, to allow radiology enough time to compile the film packets ready for the clinic.

Reporting Functions

These are functions that are utilised by radiologists and reporting radiographers. The exact way in which they are used will depend upon the nature of reporting in individual departments.

For example, in a traditional reporting environment the radiologist would report onto a dictaphone, which is then sent to the secretaries for typing onto the RIS. The RIS would then create an electronic list of typed reports that the radiologist would need to check and then verify for release to the referring clinician. As this is done via user log on and electronic means it would be simple to run a report of how long it takes for the typed report to be verified. This can often be useful in the case of complaints, or to justify increasing staff levels to deal with increasing workload.

In some departments it may be possible to type reports using hotkeys or automatic dictating devices, which type the report as you speak. The most important thing is that each step of the process is identified with an individual and that the person who created the report is responsible for its final approval.

Inquiry

One pervasive problem in the NHS is the lack of a single unique identifier for patients. This can result in every department with a hospital allocating its own number. These numbers are then deposited onto the HIS, which will upload them to the RIS. The inquiry function allows the patient to be located using any number that they may have, or failing that, their name.

The new NHS number (NNN) should eventually allow every person in the country to have a unique identifier that can be used where ever they may be.

Once the patient is located the history of that patient can be viewed, along with reports and any notes made. Future orders can also be examined, but not altered from this section.

Management Reports

This is basically a database search engine that allows the user to set up a number of automatic functions that will generate reports. For example you may want to know at the end of every month how many chest x-rays have been performed for the chest clinic. The system can generate this information for you once a month. It is worth remembering that only if the information has been accurately recorded can the information generated in reports be relied upon.

System Functions

There will normally be one person dedicated to the maintenance of the RIS and the training of individuals in its use. Along with this person there will be a core of individuals trained in the maintenance of the system. In exactly the same way as a software application in a normal PC can 'freeze' it is possible for individual terminals to stop working, interface engines to stop running, or the main computer to stop communicating.

These problems require a specific set of functions to first find out what is not working and then to correct the problem. These facilities are normally only available to those with specific access, thus preventing malicious damage to the system.

It is perhaps worth mentioning manufacturer support at this point. One of the criticisms levelled at implementers of a system is that users are often not given access to the telephone number of the manufacturer in order to report faults. Often the reason for this (contrary to popular belief) is to prevent users reporting every little fault, many of which will not be related to the running of the system. Manufacturers may spend hours on a user-reported problem, only to find that the system was functioning perfectly, but that the user's local network for that part of the hospital was off line for maintenance work at the time.

Communication

Many systems come with a local email service that pops up messages when the user logs on. This can be used to advise them of important changes in protocol, advertising shifts or merely for the exchange of social information. It is a facility that helps the users to see the benefits of an electronic database immediately.

Upgrades

These are another important feature of any RIS. Any manufacturer will constantly be trying to improve its product and clauses can be built into service contracts allowing you to take advantage of upgrades. Upgrades may have only a minimal impact on the program or they may improve it significantly, which is why they are an important part of the overall system maintenance. It is also important for the systems administrator to become as active as possible in the manufacturers user groups and forums, as upgrades will often include improvements implemented by the manufacturer as a result of feedback from these groups. The system can then evolve with the needs of the users (who are most important) rather than along the lines of the programmer's vision of how a department should work.

Audit

The use of audit to assess the accuracy of any RIS is time consuming but is inevitable as human data entry can be very poor. RIS should have a tool to allow audits on data to be carried out quickly and accurately but this is often not the case.

PROBLEMS WITH RIS

Any information system is only as good as the information that is entered in to it. Your RIS is no exception. If you want to use your RIS to tell you when to order more films of a certain size then you are relying upon the staff to record precisely how many films they have used. If staff fail to input the number of repeats they perform (for fear of being "audited" and disciplined for using too many resources) then the RIS will never be able to keep track of the actual level of film.

The functionality of a RIS is greatly reduced by

the incomplete or inaccurate recording of information by those that use it. This can be a sign that the system is too intensive, requiring too much time to input data or that the staff are inappropriately trained in the importance of good data entry and the benefits that can be gained. Whatever the cause the result will be the same.

What Happens if the RIS Goes Down?

Contingency plans must be in place for a complete failure of the RIS or for what will be done during planned shutdowns for upgrades. The easiest solution is to resort to paper records that can be input and tracked retrospectively. Such downtime needs to be kept to a minimum as the amount of paper records subsequently requiring entering can build up very quickly.

The Future of RIS

Most systems are at this time moving towards graphical user interfaces (GUIs pronounced gooey). An example of a GUI is Microsoft Windows, which uses a pointing device (the mouse) to create a picture environment that can be used to carry out any functions that are required. Undoubtedly all systems will be like this in the future, and will increase in the ease with which the GUI may be manipulated to suit the individual user.

The keyboard has remained relatively unchanged for some time and the method by which we input data will undoubtedly change.

These changes will include using voice recognition systems to input textual information. This will eventually allow radiologists to dictate reports directly onto the computer screen.

RIS in general will also become a more seamless part of the wider hospital system, and will eventually seem almost identical to all other systems within the hospital. This familiarity will allow users to access information in any part of the hospital at the click of an icon.

The future may also allow the users direct access to certain parts of the RIS over the web, such as allowing them to cancel or move appointments

CONCLUSIONS

A lot can be learned from this basic explanation of a radiology information system that is transferable to other systems within the health care environment. The key points might include;

- The numerous and complex functions that are required
- User and computer interaction
- Interface issues
- Security issues
- Access issues
- Maintenance issues
- Training issues
- Accuracy of data

At almost any level the RIS is of use to a radiology department, but the largest utility can be gained if the data is as accurate as possible.

7: COMPUTED RADIOGRAPHY AND PACS

Terry Jones

INTRODUCTION

Computed radiography (CR) is fast replacing old conventional film screen combinations and daylight processing equipment because of the potential advantages offered by a digital image.

Whilst these advantages have been discussed elsewhere it may be useful to recap here.

1. Ability to magnify image without loss of image resolution (up to a maximum point)
2. Ability to change contrast and brightness of the image to suit the viewer, or to discern pathology better
3. Simultaneous viewing of the image in more than one location
4. Teaching images available at all times. Images can be retrieved to the teaching area quickly.
5. No lost images
6. Potential increase in speed of reporting

One of the major advantages is the ability to simultaneously view the image in more than one place. This means that a junior doctor and their consultant can have a meaningful discussion on the images without either party having to leave their area of work. It also enables diagnostic imaging departments to allow the image to be sent to the ward or outpatient department for the immediate treatment of the patient, whilst also retaining a copy of the image in order for it to be reported by radiologists at the earliest opportunity.

In departments that have imaging modalities spread out over a large campus, or worse over many different campus, a digital image means that a central reporting area can be set up. This will allow radiologists to report on images from all over the diverse areas from a single point. This can mean an improvement in reporting times, as a radiologist does not have to spend time driving out to a peripheral hospital in order to report, or a saving in transport costs in getting the films back to the main site. In a hospital with limited space it can also mean that individual offices for reporting are not necessary.

Films in packets take up a lot of storage space, and present a unique hazard as a combustible material. Additionally there is the cost of having staff employed to file, retrieve and collate clinic lists, although some staff are still required when the system is replaced with a digital one.

These storage type problems can be virtually eliminated by moving to digital imaging. A digital store for a major sized Trust will only take up a small "store" room type of space, and as digital storage media increases in storage capacity and reduces in cost every few years this ability to store large amounts of information in ever smaller spaces looks likely to continue.

As digital images can be safely backed up (at another site if necessary) this means that there is a much reduced risk of images being lost. There will still be a risk of images not being available to clinicians (due to PACS failure, network problems or power cuts) but this is much less than that accepted for conventional films, and any lack of availability is likely to be short term.

PACS also supports many of the requirements implicit in the IR(ME)R 2000 regulations, such as reducing unnecessary exposures simply because the previous films are lost or because the patient has been transferred from another hospital within the Trust. The ability to simultaneously view the same image in two or more locations also opens up a wealth of possibility in a multi-site (or simply large) Trust, where resources (in terms of consultants) are spread thinly, or across sites.

It may be appropriate at this stage to clarify one of the often-quoted advantages of the digital image – and that is the "no lost film" state of affairs. It must be stressed, that in a perfect world (i.e. one in which there is no human involvement) digital images would never be lost, but in the real world this is still a little way from reality. All CR (and other methods of producing a digital image) can do is to store safely ALL the images sent to it. In this respect, digital images are never lost.

However, this statement does not take into account the images that are acquired, but never sent to a digital archive (through human error or network problems at the time of archival). Nor does it take into account the incorrect patient demographics applied to the image, which make it difficult (or impossible) to retrieve that image at a later date.

In this sense, the image is lost – because it cannot be retrieved from the archive with 100% confidence that it belongs to the patient you are searching for. Obviously a mistake where the patients name is put into the unique number field, and the unique number appears in the patient name field can be retrieved and corrected with a reasonable degree of confidence, but what about Jason Oakley and Jason Oakey. A simple letter missing means that the whole image must be called into doubt. It is for this reason that each department must put into place a stringent protocol for dealing with such instances (because no matter how good your system integration and image quality assurance is, as long as there is a human involved at any stage, such errors will occur. All you can do is to try and minimise them, put in place protocols that try to limit the unnecessary re-irradiation of any patients whose images are affected in this way.

BASIC CR SET UPS

How exactly the CR system will be set up to run will depend upon the type of department that the equipment is destined to serve, and to a lesser extent the political environment in that particular department. Sample diagrams for different set ups have been included to help in the readers understanding.

Points to consider are

- Is the CR a stand only system, or is it linked into a PACS?
- Is the CR unit only going to be producing hard copy films for other departments?
- Are the images going to be soft copy only?

To give some examples; an accident and emergency (A&E) department cannot run the risk of the CR system being inoperable due to preventable failures. The main preventable failures include network disruption and power surges or a complete loss of power. Another potential source of disruption is servicing of the equipment. It is advised that when installing the CR equipment care is taken to ensure that there is not a single point of failure.

In this instance (in an A&E department) the CR system should be linked into the main hospital network to benefit from the fast transfer times and wide bandwidth provided by many top end networks. An electrical power supply linked into the Trusts own backup generator should power

all the CR equipment. In addition the CR reader should be connected to an uninterruptible power supply (UPS) to account for the slight "hiccup" in power when the emergency generator kicks in and to provide a constant stream of electrical power, devoid of any surges or spikes. This UPS should extend to cover all the other CR equipment if possible, but if this is not an option then standard power surge protectors must be used.

All CR units, such as readers, hard disks and hardcopy printers should have their own UPS to ensure that even if the Trusts generator is non-functioning images can still be acquired (utilising battery powered mobile x-ray machines) and viewed in the vicinity of the processing equipment. A simple network hub should also be available in this area to ensure that if the network is out of action (either because of the electrical disruption or some other problem), then the CR equipment can be quickly connected to this hub to continue image processing during the emergency.

This ensures that the A&E x-ray department can act in a stand-alone capacity in any event. It is perhaps one of the unexpected benefits of CR in that it allows this type of processing during an electrical problem to continue. It must be stated here that mostly the contingency plans outlined above only allow images already taken to be processed without the loss of the image. If the department is experiencing a total power cut imaging will be the last things on most peoples minds.

CR AND PACS

With any CR installation that links into a PACS the only option is to go via a Trust network. This infrastructure is vital to allow the system to expand and to reach all the potential users dotted around the Trust. This does mean that one of the main potential areas for disaster and downtime is taken out of the hands of the diagnostic imaging department, but on the other hand few imaging departments have the depth of knowledge needed to install, upgrade and maintain a complex network infrastructure.

In a general department that only produces laser film for their end users the same rules apply, but there is scope for a little leeway. For example only the CR reader needs to be supplied with a UPS (if money is limited). This will ensure that no image is lost due to a power failure when the image is being "read". The workstation can be supplied with a surge protector to avoid power surges destroying data on the disk, or causing problems with uncontrolled shutdowns. The printer only needs a surge protector because if the power fails during printing a reprint can be sent once power is restored.

In this scenario the network can be run from a hub and patch cables for minimal cost. Speed will be reduced, but it will be acceptable for most users.

The drawback to this set up is that if PACS comes along at a later stage then the stand alone system will need to be integrated in to the larger system, and many settings on the CR system may need to be changed to facilitate this. Whilst this is not impossible, it can be very time consuming, and will result in the equipment being out of action for extended periods whilst this work is actually being performed.

FUTURE PROOFING

If the person who holds the purse strings for a particular department is a forward thinking individual then CR and in particular, PACS, will be in the forefront of their plans. However, a leader who has a tendency to be a bit of a technophobe may see PACS as a step too far, and think of it as "change for change sake".

It is no secret that CR is expensive and PACS even more so. The cost of consumables is also higher than that for conventional film, which makes it vital that any business plans are carefully researched and any savings are identified and rigorously pursued.

It can also be traumatic for staff to be faced with an influx of new technology. They may see all their acquired knowledge of conventional imaging and processing vanish overnight. This can lead to reluctance to accept the new technology, and a feeling of worthlessness. This coupled with a steep learning curve can be very daunting for some individuals.

A cost not normally considered when installing CR is that of out of hours support. No one expects there to be a person on the end of a telephone at three a.m. when the conventional processor breaks down, but when CR is implemented, because this is a "computer", suddenly the users expect there to be a person able to fix any problem 24 hours a day.

Most Trusts will have some problem with financing CR and PACS purchases due to the large initial outlay. Unfortunately the returns on investment (film savings, chemical costs etc) can take up to five years to be realised, and during this time costs may very well be higher than normal due to the dual running that is often necessary during the change over period. This emphasises the need to be vigilant in your calculations and development of business cases to ensure that all individuals are aware of the potential savings that will be made at this later date.

In some radiology departments there will be a vocal figure who is either for or against the new technology. This person may be able to sway opinion in their favour because of their influence.

In general it is found that in many departments the radiologists tend to fall into two categories with regard to computer technology in imaging – the enthusiastic and the doubters. Often the doubters will roll out the old arguments about computers never helping, and causing more work – but how many of these would welcome a change back to using a typewriter to generate reports?

Often it is the implementation and follow-up support from a company that can mean the difference between a new technology being a failure or a success.

It is also worth mentioning that the needs of a radiologist are very different from that of a clinician in a busy clinic. It is not uncommon for a radiologist to be reporting on an image in a reporting session, and realise there are (or should be) old images for that particular patient available to them. In this instance the radiologist requests these images – and is prepared to wait the 3 to 5 days it will take to retrieve these images for them. Once the images are found it is then that the report is dictated, but the newest images can now be up to a week old. For these individuals the time taken to retrieve the images is not seen as being a problem.

Now compare the experience of an orthopaedic surgeon who is in the middle of a busy clinic. If a patient arrives without the relevant images this can mean a wasted consultation, an unwarranted re x-ray to get some benefit from the appointment and a lot of aggravation. Obviously in this instance waiting three to five days is not an option − but seeing another patient whilst the old images are reloaded onto the CR system is. Thus we can see a benefit to users outside radiology that may not be apparent to those within radiology. Unfortunately this can cause resentment in that it will be seen as radiology "funding" improvements in the other department!

In many departments the finances will be controlled by a combination of people, the Assistant General Manager (AGM) and radiologists through the Assistant Clinical Director (ACD). Sometimes it is the radiologist who decides upon the equipment, the AGM who assesses the fundability of the chosen option from within existing revenue streams, and then finance who are asked to come up with inventive ways to pay for the equipment!

DIAGRAMS ILLUSTRATING VARIOUS METHODS OF CONNECTING CR EQUIPMENT

CR layout 1

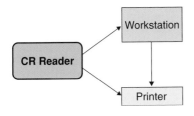

Figure 1 − Stand Alone CR Set Up

In Figure 1 the CR unit is acting simply as a means to produce a hard copy image, or film, much like a conventional processor.

Reporting would have to be done via the hard copies produced.

There is no network present to allow images to be sent to other locations, and so limits the benefits this type of set up is able to achieve.

The most obvious benefit would be the elimination of rejected images requiring "print out". These could be left on the workstation, and once the departmental reject analysis had been performed upon them, deleted forever.

CR layout 2

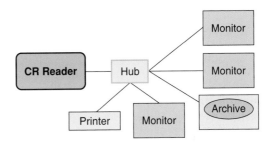

Figure 2 − Localised CR network

In figure 2, the CR reader and all other units are linked via a hub (or simple network). It allows images to be sent and shared with other devices on this limited network, and offers the opportunity to remove the hub and link direct to a main hospital network at a later date.

It also offers the first opportunity to introduce a simple archive. This can be a single disk unit that requires a lot of manual intervention to "run", and results in a library of disks being generated that must be stored as an off line library.

In this example, some reporting could be done from the monitors, as long as the reporting was done in a timely enough fashion to ensure that the images stored on the local hard disks of the remote monitors were not deleted as the disk reached and then exceeded capacity.

If there is an archive attached, then this is not such a major consideration as manually recalled images can be pulled from the archive and resent as many times as required to whichever workstation requires them. This type of set up is suited mainly for A&E departments were there is a limited requirement for old images to be available for reporting, and where fast turn around times for reported images is encouraged.

CR layout 3

In this example, we have 2 departments. Each has their own CR reader and quality assurance

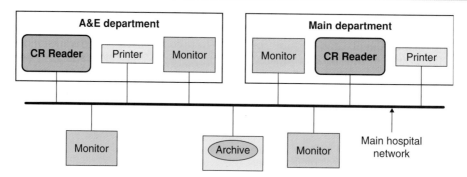

Figure 3 – Networked CR

monitor, but both are connected via the main hospital network. The archive is shared (reducing costs, whilst allowing images from both departments to be stored in a central location). More reporting can be done from the monitors increasing the value of this set up.

Please note that the printers are shown placed inside each of these departments. They are connected to the network and so it is possible to send images to print to either of these printers from any of the quality assurance stations in place, adding another level of redundancy to both these departments. Should maintenance be needed on either, the department could continue to function – simply printing their images to the other, functioning, printer.

Obviously this does require the manual retrieval of all the printed images, but this can be achieved using other ancillary staff – allowing the radiographers to continue acquiring images in the busy clinic without having to move the whole of the clinic to a different location.

CR layout 4

In figure 4 we are starting to get into the realms of PACS. Images are still only acquired using CR,

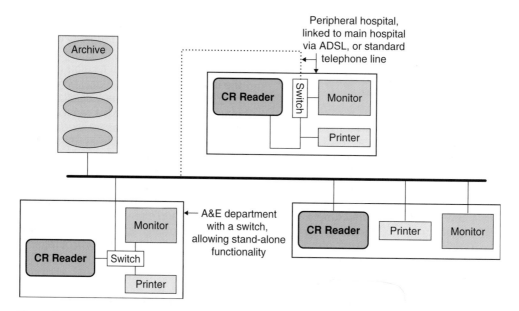

Figure 4 – Complex Network

but they are now being shared with other departments via networks. This opens up the possibility of the reporting from peripheral sites being done at a central location, with the images being routed via the network (or telephone lines if image volumes are small).

The archive can still be a single disk unit, but in this scenario it would make more sense for it to be a "jukebox" type archive – with more disks stored within the unit, meaning less human intervention in managing the retrieval of images.

NETWORK DEPENDENCY AND CONTINGENCY PLANS

One of the things common to all digital imaging modalities is that they require a network to function. This can also be their Achilles' heel. If the network is cut (due to upgrade, power failure or some other factor such as a clumsy workman physically cutting through the wires) then this effectively means you are unable to process your images.

One of the first considerations for anyone setting up a CR system in any busy department is to ensure that there is a back up plan (normally involving a stand-alone network hub or switch) for such eventualities.

The back up plans at the Author's Trust include:

- All CR units and workstations in the A&E processing area having a UPS fitted. This ensures that any power problems are covered for up to 30 minutes.
- The network switch to the main hospital network is also connected to a UPS to ensure that this continues to function in the event of power problems. Obviously if the power to switches outside this area is non existent then the switch is unable to communicate outside the confines of the A&E processing area but the equipment connected to that switch can function as normal. This means that even if we are unable to send soft copy images to clinicians we can print them to laser film in the processing area.

- A small network hub is also stored in a locked cupboard in case it is the switch itself that is faulty. This means that the hub can replace the switch to allow processing and printing to continue whilst the problem with the switch is rectified.
- There are also two CR readers, 3 naming devices (one for each x-ray room and one for the viewing area), 2 image quality assessment monitors and 2 printers to ensure that there is no single point of failure.

The above also allows us to have routine maintenance carried out on the component parts with little disruption to the running of the department, and ensure the department can continue to provide diagnostic images to A&E in any event.

PACS NETWORK REQUIREMENTS

A PACS requires a network that is far more extensive and resilient than a single CR modality, but the basic principles are the same.

SOLUTIONS TO DIFFERENT SCENARIOS

Let us now consider several different scenarios and potential solutions to them

Scenario 1
Is the CR a stand only system, or is it linked into a PACS?

Stand Alone
A stand-alone system can be used as a direct replacement for a conventional processor. A CR reader is installed, connected to a quality control workstation and printer via simple network hub and patch cables. This will allow images to be printed for use in clinics or reporting. This can be expanded slightly if radiologists decide they want to view images as soft copy, as a reporting workstation can be linked into this basic network, providing the distance between the quality control workstation and the reporting workstation is not too great (under 7 metres is preferable).

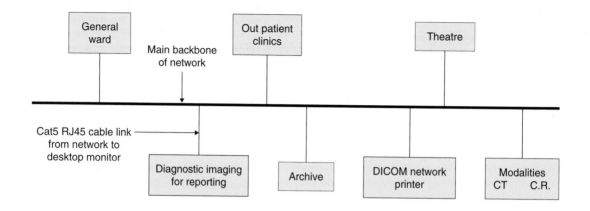

Figure 5 – Diagram of Hospital network

Linked to PACS

If the CR unit is designed to feed images into a PACS, the only solution available to you is to link into the main hospital network. This has the advantage that the network is likely to be robust, fast and have links to all the departments within the Trust. Support will be available from your Information Management and Technology (IM&T) department, and any problems with the system can be referred to them.

This means that the equipment manufacturer has to comply with the Trusts own network identification rules and only use IP addresses (Internet Protocol) supplied direct from the Trust. Problems with duplicate IP addresses should therefore, not be a factor, and should ensure that all modalities are configured in the way that the Trust is most happy with.

Any additional modalities that are acquired by the Trust can then be joined into this growing network as and when required.

Scenario 2

Is the CR unit producing films for other departments?

If you are not linking into a PACS, then you can set up a simple network to serve the local area of the CR equipment. [This can also be part of the deal with the supplier of your CR equipment (who will set up the network and maintain it (at a cost).]

This may mean that the supplier will set up the IP addresses as per their company policy. This could be a problem if you want to link this equipment into the PACS at a later date, as all these settings will need to be changed before you can join the main network of your hospital. Perhaps it is advisable here to find out the IP naming strategy for your Trust and follow this even if you are running the devices on a standalone network in the short term.

All that is required is a simple hub or switch. These are inexpensive and will allow the equipment to communicate. The downside is that the transfer of images between the various devices will be much slower than that achievable using a fast purpose designed main hospital network.

Adding other pieces of CR equipment (a radiologist reporting workstation or an archive for example) can expand this type of simple set up. The main limitation in this type of set up is the distance from the hub that each piece of equipment is located. As you will be using simple cat5 RJ45 connectors to join the equipment to the hub a limiting factor of 3 meters (but some cables will run to 30 metres if a decrease in speed is accepted) is applicable.

If there is a need to expand to a larger number of network devices than the number of slots available on the hub being used it is likely that the requirement exists to join a dedicated network.

Scenario 3

Are the images going to be soft copy only?

If the images are for a purely electronic environment then using a stand-alone network is not advisable. In this instance speed is of importance and a dedicated fast network should be utilised to cope with the demand placed upon the system by the large file sizes.

In addition a soft copy only environment is by definition one where clinicians other than radiologists can view images, and in this case there will be a need to have your main hospital information system as well as the RIS integrated with the image system (or put simply - a full PACS)

INFORMATION FLOWS

The information flow for a basic CR system is

- Patient arrives with x-ray request.
- Request verified as appropriate and booked onto the RIS.
- Patient demographics input into CR system.
- Image taken and processed.
- Image and patient demographics attached (DICOM) forever.
- Image either sent to be viewed on another monitor or printed (sometimes both).

In a CR system there is a need to get the demographics of the patient onto the image. In an ideal world all of the information systems in the hospital would be integrated with one another and there would be a common unique patient identifier that every department would use (such as the new NHS number).

This would then be electronically up-loaded into the CR system from the radiology information system (RIS), or direct from the main hospital patient master index (PMI). This has the advantage of maintaining patient data integrity by reducing the chance for operator error in spelling the patient name. Unfortunately this is achieved at a cost. In many stand only CR systems (or other digital modalities for that matter) the cost equation between integrating the modality in question to the RIS or not is often too prohibitive. This means that the radiographer has to manually enter the demographics at the time of examination, which can lead to errors in data integrity, is time consuming but has little "visible" cost to the organisation.

If a stand-alone system is in use there can still be gains made if the radiologists are using a monitor to report. The film that is printed can go back to the referring clinician with the patient, whilst the electronic image is sent for radiologist reporting on the dedicated monitors in radiology.

MINI PACS OR FULL PACS

A question often asked is what is the difference between mini PACS and full PACS.

The PACS aspect is easy – this is the ability to view old and new electronic images simultaneously on a computer monitor. I do not know if there is an official DICOM definition of full and mini PACS, but how I like to describe the difference is that a full PACS has many different modalities able to be viewed on the multiple monitors. There is also integration with the RIS to allow for the electronic transfer of patient demographics between the PACS, modalities and the RIS. The retrieval of historical images is also likely to be automatic – with triggers from either the RIS or better still from both the RIS and the Hospital Information System (HIS). Using the HIS means that patients using the hospital for non radiological consultations will still have their old radiological images retrieved from long term store to RAID, in case their images are required in clinic.

In a mini PACS there is likely to be a single modality supplying images to the monitors, and integration to the RIS is probably not evident. This means that a mini PACS is likely to be a manual affair – with human interaction needed to ensure old images are available at the same time as the newly acquired.

A mini PACS can be a useful tool in a small department, as well as an A&E or orthopaedic unit within a bigger hospital. It is also able to metamorphose into a full-blown PACS when resources allow.

One of the best reasons for starting with a mini PACS is that you can build up a back library of images. This means that when the department changes over to a full PACS at a later stage the disruption to other departments encountered by having to run a film system alongside a soft copy system is minimised. Obviously there are images that will pre date the mini PACS but the majority of patients seen in many clinics can be moved from film to electronic images relatively easily.

ARCHIVING MEDIA CONSIDERATIONS

As mentioned in other chapters there are many different types of archival media (see Chapter Three – Equipment).

Probably the best known and widely used is magento-optical disk (MOD). In a WORM disk the image can be written and then never changed. Any subsequent retrieval of the image will result in the image appearing exactly as it was at the time of committal to archive.

MOD media are established, relatively cheap and readily available. They are also robust and slim, making them ideal for single disk archives or for more elaborate multi disk jukeboxes that still retain an element of off line storage. Once standing side by side the disks take up a small amount of space, meaning they can be accommodated close to the disk unit for quicker retrieval times.

Floppy disks and CD-R are also theoretically possible as storage media – but the relatively small capacities of both of these media means they are not suitable as a long-term storage option.

A floppy disk (1.44MB capacity) would only be able to store about three images from a computed tomography (CT) head scan, and CT images are one of the smallest file sizes from the DICOM standard equipment. So this option is not one that should be given any serious thought.

A CD-R would be better able to cope with larger file sizes, but again the image volumes generated by most imaging departments would soon overwhelm an archive running on CD-R. It may be possible to burn a patient's most recent examination on CD-R to allow transfer of the images to another DICOM hospital.

Another archive media that may be feasible in a small department may be a standard computer hard disk. With disk sizes now available in 60GB and above these may provide an option

for archiving a small departments (or vetinary practise) images for several months. With a simple network set-up more disks could be added to this archive as needs required – but this system is fraught with database issues and maintenance problems and so should be viewed as ramblings for the time being.

The main contender to replace the MOD for long term archiving is the Digital Versatile Disk (DVD).

DVD can store many gigabytes of image information at present. They are easy to manufacture and are likely to increase their capacity as technology advances. DVD's offer all the same advantages as MOD plus a few unique to DVD. They are ultra slim, easy to store and cheaper than MOD in most instances. DVDs are also used and accepted in the entertainment industry, which tends to mean they will be around for a long time and that prices will come down as more people utilise this form of media.

COMPRESSION

One of the most important questions that must be asked when you consider archival (after what media to use) is what level of compression you are prepared to accept on that image?

Compression is a means to reduce the image file size, meaning less space is used when you store it. However, the act of compression also causes the detail in the image to suffer.

The two most common terms any radiographer is likely to hear describing compression are lossy and lossless. Both these methods of compression are allowed within the DICOM standard, and the main difference between them is the amount of image degradation that takes place.

Lossy can reduce the storage requirement by up to 30 times of that occupied by the original. This may, at first glance, appear to offer much to a PACS. If the image file size is 30 times less, then the time it takes for that image to be transmitted from A to B via the network will also be less (meaning the image appears on screen faster). It also means that instead of replacing a MOD (or whatever storage media you are using) every day you could replace it every 30 days – a significant financial incentive.

However, as always, nothing in life is for free and the price paid for using lossey compression (especially at 30 times) is the resulting degradation in image quality. A CR image compressed by this factor would exhibit image artefacts making the resultant image unsuitable for front line reporting.

The only potential use for this type of compression is for consultations at GP surgeries or out patient clinics, where the primary aim of the image is to show the patient the general impression of what their particular problem is.

Lossless compression can reduce the storage requirement of the original image by a maximum factor of 2.5. This is achieved with no reduction in quality of the original image. This makes it ideal for use in PACS and is often used in the long-term, secure storage area of the PACS. This has the effect of making retrieval of the images from this area slightly faster but also helps to keep the cost of providing consumables (in terms of storage disks) down.

The RAID (Random Array of Interchangeable Disks, another name for the short term store) is often set with no compression factor at all, meaning that for reporting all images will be in their original state.

The dangers of archiving, the level of compression and not archiving at all will have to be weighed up.

WHEN TO ARCHIVE

Another consideration you will face is when to archive the images you have acquired. By archive, we mean writing the images to non-erasable media.

It is a fact that most CR systems come with a substantial hard disk, which means that several days worth of images can be stored locally. In fact most modern diagnostic equipment that has a DICOM component will also have some form of local hard drive on which to store images.

Having an image existing in only one place is dangerous. If you are unable to retrieve from that location (for a variety of reasons - including servicing) then the image is in fact lost to you (at least for that short period). It is sensible to move the image to a second, more secure area as soon as possible. In a PACS situation you have the local hard disk, the RAID and the long term

secure store. The RAID is in fact a collection of hard disks that have a controller and complex software that enables the images on the storage area to be rebuilt if one or more of the hard disks fails. This means that the most common cause for concern is removed (hard disk failure), making the RAID a very secure place for images to be stored.

It is not feasible (in terms of money and foot print size) to have a RAID as your long term store – so the RAID sends images to be stored on some form of removable media (MOD disk normally) elsewhere. By doing this you are also adding another layer of resilience into the system. It is at this point that most PACS will stop – but the system could also send the image to a second long-term store off the actual site – which means that you are then covered in case of a catastrophic event on the site of the PACS archive. Most departments setting up a PACS will opt not to do this for financial reasons, but it should be considered.

It is apparent that storing the images on the local hard disk is not the ideal solution to long term storage. So when should archiving take place?

Firstly there will be a difference between full PACS and mini PACS.

With full PACS there will be a RAID (which means you have the ability to change the look of the image or correct demographic errors). With a mini PACS there is often no RAID and the images go straight to a long term, unalterable store.

With full PACS the answer is relatively simple in that the user sends the images to RAID as soon as they are quality checked at the workstation of the modality they are working on. There is still a second chance to change the information on the RAID (should the need arise) but the volume of image traffic being dealt with by the RAID is kept to a steady, and therefore manageable level as the system is, in effect, trickle feeding images throughout the day.

If the system is set-up to send all of the images acquired during a clinic (or from a particular modality) in one job lot, this would put a huge strain on even the most robust networks. The RAID would also struggle meaning that the whole system would slow down whilst the influx of work was dealt with. This is not an ideal situation and can be eliminated by trickle feeding images as they are approved by the radiographer at each modality.

If your facility is using a PACS to allow clinicians to view the images as soft copy then it also makes sense to make them available on the system as soon as possible so that the patients management can be reviewed.

In a mini PACS there is no RAID – and yet there is still the problem of images being lost or inaccessible. In most CR systems there is an option to send images direct from the reader to the long-term store before quality assurance is undertaken. This is a double-edged sword – on the one hand you have every image taken stored safely, but this means all your demographic errors and rejects are also recorded forever and you will have to implement policies to deal with these human errors. This also means that any image recalled from this archive needs to be checked again by a radiographer before being allowed out for general viewing (because it was stored straight from the CR reader, this image has not been approved prior to storage).

Alternatively, even if the image is incorrectly named, you can (in theory at least) be safe in the knowledge that the image is "somewhere" in your archive.

However if you choose the mini PACS to commit your image to long term store after the image has been quality checked you can reduce the burden of your long term store, and ensure that all images are stored at their optimum. In this case you remove the automatic element (sending image direct from CR reader) and you introduce the human aspect. If you forget to send the approved images to long-term store you end up with no record of that particular examination.

As this is a catch 22 situation each department must judge how best to approach this problem based on their knowledge of the staff base at that particular department.

In my Trust I have both scenarios in existence, and I can honestly say I have not solved the riddle as I have problems with both!

ELECTRONIC PATIENT RECORD

PACS is a major component of the EPR, and as such it is a good idea if your electronic archive is

started as soon as possible. The sooner images are acquired and stored in a recognised industry format the sooner you can stop running dual systems in the future.

PROBLEMS WITH CR

At this point it is appropriate to take a moment to discuss the darker side of CR.

Whilst there are numerous articles extolling the virtue of CR, and it can honestly be said that those with CR would not go back to conventional after using CR, there are problems that are unique to this new technology.

Some of these are general computer problems, such as less technically minded members of staff not understanding how to use a mouse or common terms such as "left click". Others are issues that have raised their heads after implementation and can be something of a surprise.

This section will share some of these problems – both as a warning and also as a indication that no matter how well prepared you are, there will still be things that have to be dealt with by "fire fighting" as they occur.

1. CR is not an extension of conventional processing

In the author's Trust the mistake was made of thinking CR was simply an evolution of conventional processing. The same equipment was used to "take" the x-rays, and the new technology simply changed the manner in which the images were processed.

This was wrong on many levels. CR should be viewed as a different modality that requires a return to the drawing board before use. How many departments change CT scanners without a corresponding "this is how to use it" period?

CR also requires things to be done in sequence. It is a computer and does not exhibit any intelligence of it's own. If you make a mistake in CR because you were busy the CR does not assess the situation and say "I am sure that is wrong, so I'll correct it". This also applies to name errors – in electronic imaging you cannot stick a white label with the correct patient details on the corner of the image.

CR also has it's own technique. For example one third of the image plate must be covered, and collimation must be perfect. If these "rules" are not followed the resultant image will require some manipulation at the workstation to allow them to be viewed optimally.

2. Exposure

CR is not like conventional imaging where exposure is concerned. Whilst it is true that CR can deal with lower exposures than conventional (but only marginally), and the resultant image can be manipulated to look acceptable, the level of detail in this image is the same for both. CR is just better at hiding slight exposure errors.

It is also important that the staff within the department are made aware that a "black" CR image is not necessarily overexposed! A continuing problem is explaining to radiographers (who are still "conventional processors" at heart) that reducing the exposure on a black (apparently over exposed) CR image will not make the image better. You need to manipulate electronically or change the manner in which it was acquired (cover a third of the cassette, reduce scatter etc) rather than lower the exposure. Always check the sensitivity values of an image prior to any retakes.

CR also likes quantity rather than quality in terms of exposure. This means that an image acquired with a high kVp and low mAs will not be as good as one acquired with a kVp adequate for the body part and a corresponding adequate mAs. This is often anathema to radiographers who want to use high kVp to reduce the dose to patient (at cost of contrast). If you want to display a low contrast CR image – simply adjust the display factors to achieve this, but use a reasonable mAs to acquire the image in the first place.

CR allows you to aquire a perfect image and then let every viewer manipulate it electronically to their idea of the perfect image.

3. Out of hours support

It came as a surprise to the trust that radiographers who would not expect 24-hour support for a conventional processor did expect this with the CR equivalent. It may be that the introduction of a computer also introduces expectation that the computer will be supported at all times, or perhaps it is the fact that most radiographers can pull apart and solve many processor problems but have no idea of how to solve even simple computer issues.

Perhaps this removal of the skills acquired in dealing with processor problems has created the expectation that because you are unable to solve the problem on the ground – there is someone who will. Whatever the reason – expect to be in the position where 24 hour support for the CR system is expected by the users. In most instances this support is simply explaining how to resolve a simple "computer freeze", and this can be done over the phone in minutes, meaning that the department is out of action for the shortest possible time. If manufacturer support is the only option, then this simple problem would be left until the next working day (which is a long time if the system froze at 6pm on Friday!).

Most CR manufacturers will not offer 24 hour support (it would be too expensive for the department – and response times would be unavoidably long). The result is likely to be a few "superusers" providing this support, but it is unfair to expect this 24 hour commitment without appropriate remuneration.

4. Reprints

One of the more useful aspects of an electronic image is that it can be printed as many times as is necessary. Obviously this should only be the single time that is the equivalent of the conventional. However, a patient whose images are "lost" and are now in the hospital for a consultation can have their images reprinted and sent to that clinic very quickly. On the surface this can be seen as a very useful function.

However, this is not all good news. If an image is reprinted the department incurs extra cost. This cost may be offset against the time it takes the film library staff to search in vain but it is worth bearing in mind this particular CR "advantage" can quickly become an expensive way to run a film library.

In the author's experience many staff now come straight to request a reprint if a film is not instantly available, as they know that the image can be printed off in minutes – guaranteed. Compare this to most film libraries that could only just match this speed in the instances when the film packet is actually in store but if the packet has already been loaned to another clinic then the search for that packet has to continue.

Requesting a reprint means that staff are away from their work area for the shortest possible time.

However, this will push the budget for printing in your department ever upward. This will require careful monitoring, and strict protocols in place to ensure that reprints are done for valid, patient centred reasons. Note that trying to exercise the free market principle of charging out patients or wards for the reprint will most likely result in failure and forests worth of angry letters from consultants in these areas!

Some of the protocols designed in the author's department include only reprinting on confirmation from your film library staff that they have failed to find any trace of the patients packet (this removes the quick lazy approach from ward or clinic staff trying to bypass the library). It is also policy to make reprinting as difficult as possible on the day of imaging (this is about the only time that the department can be 100% certain that the Imaging Department has not lost the films as they were given direct to the team caring for that patient).

5. Reporting

As odd as this sounds, reporting CR images can present it's own unique problems. This only applies if you report CR as soft copy – if you report CR for hardcopy then the normal department protocol for dealing with conventional films can be followed.

Simple things such as ensuring that the request forms arrive in the same place as the soft copy images become a challenge. Obviously this has to be manual – but the forms must be "ordered" in some way (alphabetical by date has proven the easiest way for us) to facilitate fast through put of images.

The above are just a short example of the problems that might be encountered during the implementation of a new system. Further examples of both radiographers' and radiologists' experiences can be found in Chapter Eleven – Practical Experiences.

CONCLUSION

CR is an evolution of conventional x-ray, and looks likely to be here for the foreseeable future.

Without CR many PACS systems would not be possible (it is possible to digitise all conventional images but this would be costly in terms of time and resources). PACS is proof that technology can help deliver significant patient benefits, if the Trust is prepared to invest. PACS is not cheap and in the early years it will cost more than a film-based system in purely monetary terms, but PACS and CR offers non-cash releasing savings that can often mean more to the department than money.

For example having CR images means that reprints are available at a moments notice and how much patient contact time do clinicians waste taking an x-ray to be reviewed by another specialist?

If you are thinking of, or if you have just procured a CR system it may be worthwhile stopping a moment and reflecting on a few points.

1. One of the top priorities of imaging systems is image resolution. However, with CR whilst this point is still important another factor comes into play that must be balanced with the image resolution and that is SPEED. It is no good having the best resolution CR system if the system can only cope with 1 or 2 images every few minutes. In a busy A&E department speed is essential and this must be borne in mind when writing the business case and specification for the CR.
2. Size of the CR component parts. Remember that CR is a system that comes with many parts. As a minimum there will be a naming device and a laser reader acting as a processor. Space will have to be found to accommodate these, close to network points and power sockets. A wet processor normally sits in the middle of the viewing room, and any replacement goes into the same place – but your CR reader is better placed against a wall to hide the trailing wires. The naming device will also have to be located close to the work – ideally in the imaging room, but is there enough shelf space to accommodate? Most imaging rooms are small and are always packed to the brim already.
3. Be aware that CR is computer based. This means you have all the problems associated with computers to consider.

    These problems include unexpected shut downs due to power blips, which means all

CR equipment should have a power surge protector as a minimum, but an uninterruptible power supply would be better.

Another problem is support. It is all well and good choosing a CR system, but you will have to ensure that someone from the department is available and knowledgeable enough to deal with the common computer and manufacturer specific problems on a day to day basis. It is probably unacceptable to have to wait for an engineer to call to simply reboot a computer that has crashed. Many departments think that their own I.T. will provide this support, but often the I.T. department are as short staffed as everyone else and they simply do not have the manpower to provide this type of cover – and the department would have to find the funds to pay the I.T. department for this support.

4. Out of hours support. As with the day to day support, staff expect computers to have a 24 hour on call support. Often because staff feel "lost" with computers they may feel vulnerable having to deal with a problem in the middle of the night. Pulling apart a wet processor is normal for most radiographers – but having to solve a computer problem is another matter! When writing the business case remember to include this out of hours support in the costings!

5. Clinician acceptance. It is easy to convince radiologists that CR is a move in the right direction. They are able to report on images using high resolution monitors, and as long as they can be convinced to report in a central area instead of their offices (as the monitors are too expensive to place into each radiologists office) then there is a benefit to be able to report on images as soon as they are acquired, without having to wait until the packets are returned from out patients or wards. Clinicians on the other hand have to accept the hard copy produced by the CR system, or lose their ability to use "God's own lightbox" to view films by having to move to a monitor. The monitor offers significant advantages in terms of image manipulation but removes the flexibility of the clinician in where he views the images.

6. Printing to acquisition size. Please ensure the system you choose will print an image at acquisition size once acquired on the CR system. Remember that all orthopaedic templates assume that hard copy images are "life size" – thus any deviation from this expectation will lead to an error in the size of component used in an operation. Simply stating "must print to film" in your business case is not good enough. A CR system can print an image the size of a postage stamp to film and fulfil this question – but how many clinicians would accept a 35*43cm film with a chest printed in the centre the size of a stamp! In the specifications try to word the statement to avoid such misunderstandings – such as using "acquisition size". If your CR system does not print to 100% acquisition size then ensure that your clinicians are made aware of this fact to avoid any unpleasantness later on.

Digital radiography in its many forms is here to stay but its implementation is not going to be easy. However, with good planning and an acceptance of the limitations the benefits in both cost and to patient care can be readily realised.

8: IMAGE PROCESSING

Michael Farquharson and Jason Oakley

INTRODUCTION

IMAGE REPRESENTATION: A SIMPLE MODEL

An image is a two dimensional area of varying light intensity. It can be represented by a function $f(x,y)$. The value of f at any spatial coordinate (x,y) gives the intensity, or degree of lightness/darkness of the image at that point, as shown in figure 1.

In an analogue image the value of the function is continuous and represent all degrees of intensity from black to white.

SAMPLING

For image processing, the image function $f(x,y)$ must be digitised both spatially (i.e. position) and in intensity (grey level quantisation). In other words we divide the analogue image up into squares (or a matrix) and give each square a number depending on the brightness of that square. The result of this procedure is a digital image, and each square is called a PIXEL (picture element). The matrix size is normally an integer power of two i.e.

$$M = 2^n$$

typically 512×512 or 1024×1024. The number of pixels will be a factor in determining the quality of an image. Figure 2 shows a simple example to illustrate why this occurs.

The grey level (G) given to each pixel is also governed by

$$G = 2^n$$

Usually $n = 8$ so that each pixel can have any of 256 grey levels. The number of grey levels will also be a factor in determining the quality of an image.

Figure 3 shows the same image being represented using various levels of grey level quantisation.

NYQUIST FREQUENCY

Nyquist theorem states that if you have frequency f, then in order to sample this frequency correctly the sampling frequency must be at least 2f. For example if you wish to have the equivalent resolution of 5 lp/mm then each line pair will be 0.2mm. To sample this correctly the sampling rate must be at least 0.1mm, or double the frequency that we wish to see.

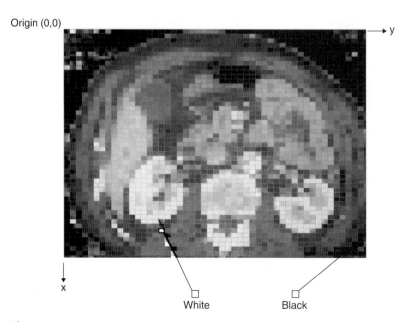

Figure 1 – Image components

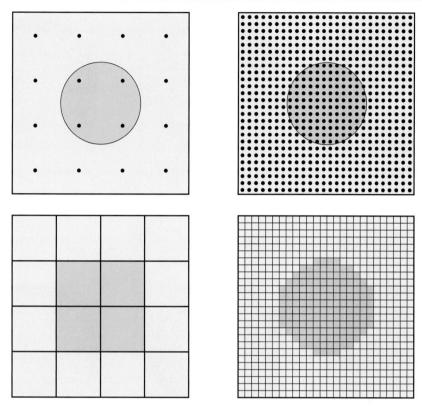

Figure 2 – The top images are shown with the sampling points. The bottom images show how the sampling rate affects the image quality

If the sampling rate is too coarse or the system is not capable of resolving such detail then an artefact can appear known as aliasing.

GREY LEVEL HISTOGRAM

A grey level histogram reflects the distribution of grey levels in the image (i.e. the number of pixels that have a given grey level between 0 and 256. Figure 4 shows a typical histogram for different types of image.

FOURIER TRANSFORMS

Any signal or waveform can be made up from the addition of a number of sine and cosine waves with varying amplitudes and frequencies.

Figure 5 shows how two cosine waves appear when added together. Consider a simple cosine function $\cos(f_0 t)$. This has a single frequency of f_0.

Note it is a function of time, we say it is in the time domain. Now consider a cosine function $\cos(2f_0 t)$. This has a frequency of $2f_0$ i.e. twice the first wave. If we add the two functions together we get a complex looking function made up of two simple ones. We can show these graphs not in the time domain but in the frequency domain as shown if figure 6.

The function $\cos(f_0 t)$ has one frequency at f_0 which is represented by a line on the frequency axis. Similarly with the function $\cos(2f_0 t)$. The added waveform however consists of two frequencies which are plotted on the frequency axis. To get from one domain to the other we carry out a Fourier transform. Almost any value that changes with time or space can be broken down in a similar manner. With an image, we can translate our spatial domain, i.e. image (x,y) into a frequency domain (called K space) via a Fourier transform. Similarly we can convert from the frequency domain back to the spatial domain using an inverse Fourier transform.

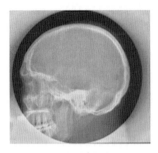

a) 8 bit - 256 grey levels

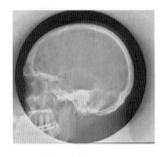

b) 7 bit - 128 grey levels

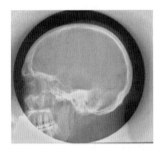

c) 6 bit - 64 grey levels

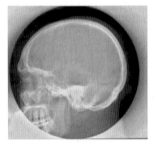

d) 5 bit - 32 grey levels

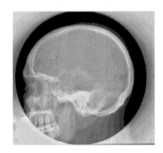

e) 4 bit - 16 grey levels

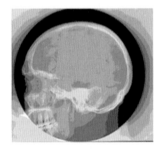

f) 3 bit - 8 grey levels

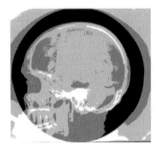

g) 2 bit - 4 grey levels

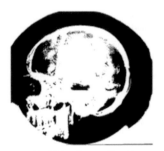

h) 1 bit - 2 grey levels

Figure 3 – Effect of varying bit depth and therefore number of grey levels

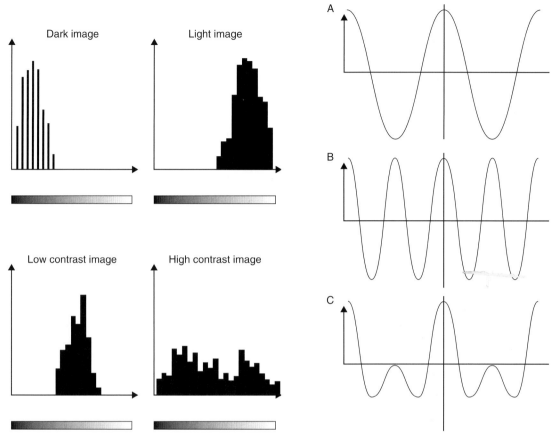

Figure 4 – Typical histograms for dark and light images and high and low contrast images

Figure 5 – A complicated function, (c) is made up from the addition of two simple cosine functions

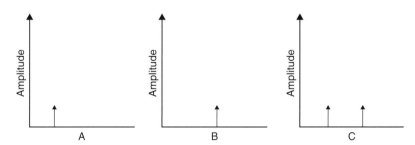

Figure 6 – The functions in figure 5 are shown here in the frequency domain

IMAGE ENHANCEMENT

We may want to carry out certain processes on an image to make it more suitable for a specific application. We can use both spatial domain methods and frequency domain methods. The spatial domain is the image plane itself with direct manipulation of pixels in the image. The frequency domain processing is based on the manipulation of the Fourier transform of the image.

SPATIAL DOMAIN METHODS

Consider the spatially varying intensity function (image) f(x,y). The processed image can be expressed as

$$G(x,y) = T\,[f(x,y)]$$

where T is some form of operator. The main approach is to define a neighbourhood about a target pixel (x,y) called a mask, template, window or filter.

Point operations

In point operations, a new grey level for each pixel in an image is calculated from its original grey level. One pixel is worked on at a time. Typical applications are inverting an image i.e positive to negative, contrast stretching (or windowing).

Arithmetic operations on two images.

1) Point operations permit us to combine two or more images pixel by pixel.
2) If we take the mean of the pixel values from several images we will help to minimise noise, as illustrated in figure 7.

The complementary operation is to subtract two images as illustrated in figure 8.

This is used in medical applications e.g. DSA. An image is aquired with no contrast media present, then with contrast present. A subtraction is made and we are left with images of contrast only.

HISTOGRAM EQUALISATION

Consider the image shown in figure 9, along with its histogram. We can see from the histogram that the image is predominantly a dark one. (if 0 is black and 255 is white) .

To enhance this image and to use the full range of grey levels we amplify the original levels (GL_{in}) using the formula

$$GL_{out} = GAIN \times GL_{in} + BIAS$$

The GAIN is defined by the user while the BIAS is determined by the mean grey level of the original image and the mean grey level of the desired output image using;

$$BIAS = MEAN_{out} - Gain \times MEAN_{in}$$

The $MEAN_{in}$ of the image in this case is 92 and if we want a $MEAN_{out}$ of say 150 and a GAIN of 1.5, the relationship between the input and output grey levels is

$$GL_{out} = 1.5 \times GL_{in} + 12$$

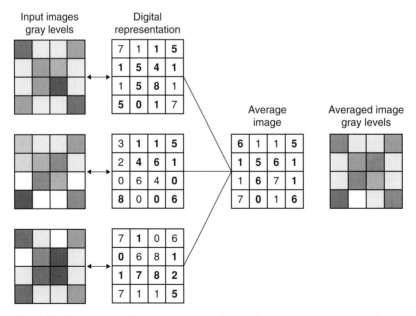

Figure 7 – The mean of the pixel value, (x,y) in each image is calculated and mapped to the new output image

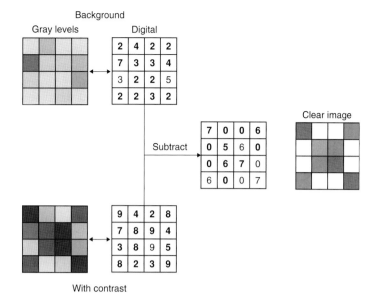

Figure 8 – Digital subtraction via a point operation.

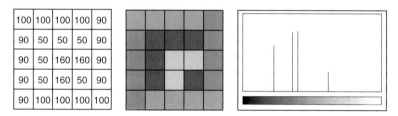

Figure 9 – Prior to histogram equalisation

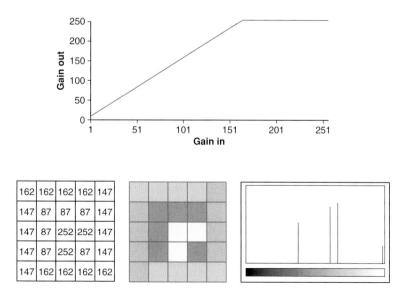

Figure 10 – After histogram equalisation

This is the formula for a straight line graph (i.e. $y = mx + c$), hence our look up table (LUT) will look like that shown in figure 10. We now apply this to each pixel in the image, which will result in the modified image and histogram.

Local Operations

The aim of local operations is to emphasise or suppress the grey level patterns around a certain pixel.

SPATIAL FILTERING

A chosen algorithm will process defined pixels around a central pixel in the input image. The result is a new grey level, which is assigned to the current pixel in the output image. The "mask" is now shifted one pixel to right and the calculation repeated. This is carried out row by row. Figure 11 shows such an operation using a 3×3 pixel mask to smooth noise in an image. The mean value of the pixels is found and mapped to the output image.

Note that the border pixels of the image are never reached hence the image shrinks. This is not normally a problem. Border pixels can be given the value 0 by initially setting all pixels in the output image to zero.

GREY LEVEL SMOOTHING

The above example was called a mean operation and tends to blur out the noise of an image but also the data. An alternative is the weighted mean in which the grey levels in the mask are multiplied by a certain weight or coefficient. Figure 12 shows the masks for the mean operator and a weighted mean operator.

The weighted mean mask gives more emphasis on the central pixel but still blurs image.

Other alternatives are the min operator which cleans dark areas of an image and max operators which clean light areas of an image. A combination of all these which cleans the entire image without blurring is the median operator. As an example, take a 3×3 mask and look at the values in the pixels. These are then sorted in numerical order and the output pixel assigned the median value as shown in figure 13.

Note there are many algorithms that can be employed and many filters. Low pass filters

attenuate or eliminate the high frequency components while leaving the low frequencies untouched. High frequency components characterise edges and sharp details in an image so a low pass filter will blur the image. High pass filters eliminate low frequencies, which characterise the slowly varying characteristics of an image i.e. overall intensity and contrast. High pass filters result in the sharpening of edges in an image. Band pass filters are used to remove selected frequencies from the image.

Global Operations. (Frequency domain methods)

Global operations require that we use all the pixels in the input image to calculate the grey level for one output pixel. Main use is the Fourier transform. The basic procedure is shown;

Why are we bothering to do a Fourier transform? The reason is we can manipulate the image in frequency space and then convert back to real image. Mathematically we are doing the following

$$G(u,v) = H(u,v)F(u,v)$$

where $F(u,v)$ is the Fourier transform of an image. We need to find a suitable transfer function $H(u,v)$ that will gives us our desired modification $G(u,v)$ which can be inverse Fourier transformed to the final image. An example of this might be to remove certain frequencies from the image to remove noise or enhance edges etc. Consider a high and low pass filter.

The ideal high pass filter can be thought of as having a threshold frequency above which the frequencies are kept and below which the frequencies are removed. This is illustrated in figure 14.

Note that we are showing the image in frequency or K space. Low frequencies are in the middle of K space whereas high frequencies are at the edges. In K space therefore we would remove all frequencies below the threshold.

The ideal low pass filter can be thought of as the opposite of the high pass as shown in figure 15. Note in K space we removed the frequencies from the edges i.e. high frequencies.

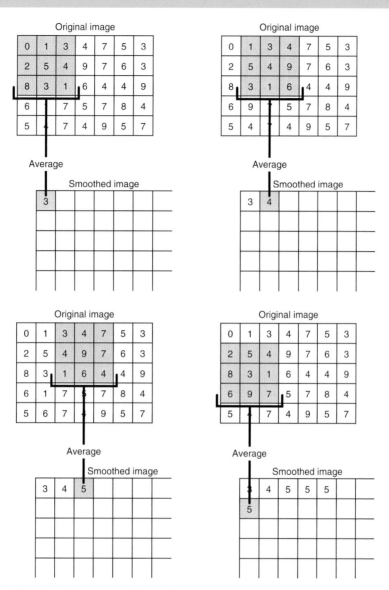

Figure 11 – Image smoothing using a local operator

Smoothing masks

Mean

1	1	1
1	1	1
1	1	1

Weighted mean

1	2	1
2	4	2
1	2	1

Figure 12 – Mean and weighted mean operator masks

IMAGE SEGMENTATION

Image segmentation means subtracting an object from its background or subdividing an image into its constituent parts or objects

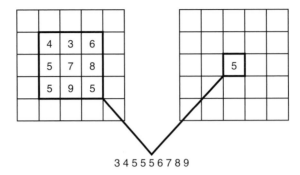

Figure 13 – The median operator.

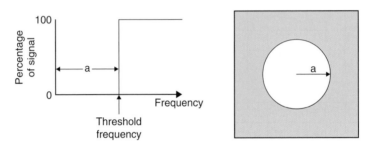

Figure 14 – High pass filtering

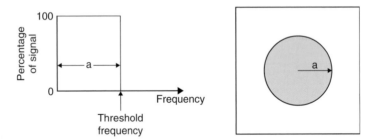

Figure 15 – Low pass filtering

Region Orientated Segmentation: Thresholding

Consider an image with two distinguishable grey levels. The histogram of the image will show the difference between the grey levels. We can place a threshold between the two main regions and label all pixels below with "0" and all above with 1. This will create a black and white image as shown in figure 16. The pixels with the same number are now "connected" so shapes can be determined. It is now easier to describe certain features on the image i.e. area of shapes, perimeter distances etc.

Detection of discontinuities e.g. points lines and edges.

The detection of such properties are normally achieved by running a mask through the image. The mask shown in figure 17 will easily detect points. It is the sum of the products that is given to the new pixel. If this value is greater than a set threshold we can say we have found a point.

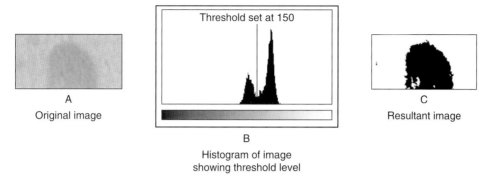

A
Original image

Threshold set at 150

B
Histogram of image
showing threshold level

C
Resultant image

Figure 16 – Thresholding

−1	−1	−1
−1	8	−1
−1	−1	−1

Figure 17 – A mask used to detect points

Line detection may utilise similar masks.

Edge detection is very important in image analysis where an edge is the change in grey levels between two objects. The process, shown in figure 18, is based on a derivative operator.

Note the profile is not abrupt because digital transitions between the grey levels are blurred. The first derivative curve is positive at the leading edge and negative at the trailing edge for the first image, and opposite for the second image. The second derivative is positive for the dark side of the edge and negative for the light side and zero for constant grey levels. The first derivative can be used to find an edge and the sign of the second derivative used to determine if the pixel is on the dark or light side of the edge.

The techniques described should yield a set of pixels that lie on a boundary. In reality this set of pixels is seldom complete because of noise, and breaks in boundaries. To overcome this, the pixels found by edge detection are linked via a linking algorithm.

Contour orientated segmentation

A series of steps are carried out in this procedure.

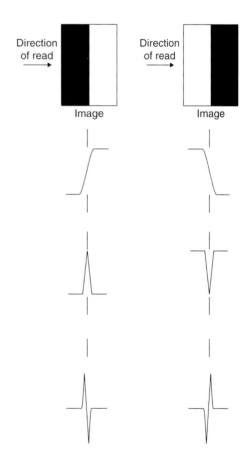

Figure 18 – Edge Detection

1. Detection of contour points

We need to enhance the grey level differences in image. This is carried out using a gradient operator which finds the size and direction of the changes.

2. Contour Enhancement

The gradient operator results in a contour with a ridge profile due to the smoothing action of the operator as shown in figure 19.

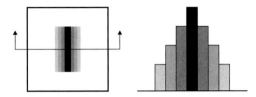

Figure 19 – The gradient operator

The peak pixels that have the highest gradient magnitudes are most likely to represent the actual location of the contour. A process known as thinning can remove the pixels on each side of the summit. This leaves a line of one pixel width around each contour.

3. Linking contour points

Some form of analysis is now needed which collects connected contour points, a process called contour linking is used that provides a list of the co-ordinates of each summit pixel.

4. Contour Approximation

An algorithm is now used to approximate the segments represented by the contours

THE HOUGH TRANSFORM

This is a form of contour oriented segmentation with some special properties.

Consider a straight line, which can be defined by the formula

$$y = mx + c$$

Another description is in polar co-ordinates and uses the perpendicular distance r to the origin and the angle θ between r and the x-axis (as shown if figure 20).

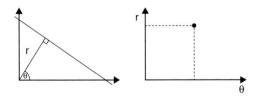

Figure 20 – Polar coordinates

These descriptions are linked via the formula.

$$r = x \cos\theta + y \sin\theta$$

Assume we have a thinned gradient image obtain as previously described and shown in figure 21.

The arrows are contour points that lie on a straight line and have magnitude and a direction. The task is for the computer to recognise this as a straight line and can achieve this via a Hough Transform.

We know the x,y co-ordinates of the contour points and from this we can calculate that $\theta = 45$ degrees. From this data we can easily calculate that r = 40. We can now plot this in the r, θ domain (given the name *accumulator*). Since there are 6 r contour points in this example, the number 6 goes into the accumulator.

When this has been carried out for all contour points in the image we have to analyse the accumulator. Each of the accumulator cells that have a value greater than 1 represent at least 2 contour points on a straight line. Consider a 128 by 128 image as shown. The line must cross the x and y axis i.e. x = o at some point, so we can calculate y as we know r and θ. Similarly for x. In this case it comes out to be 56 for both x and y because we have a 45 degree line.

COMPRESSION

INTRODUCTION

The techniques of data compression have been around for some time, primarily driven by the initial limited storage capacity of storage devices. However as storage capacity has expanded other reasons have become apparent. Whilst storage has become cheaper, the time it takes to transfer a file is now an issue, and there is much debate over the speed of Internet and network access.

But whilst storage costs are being reduced and transfer times are increasing, medical radiology is creating more data that will need to be transferred, hence if an appropriate compression algorithm can be found then it is sensible to use it to either reduce storage costs or increase the amount of data that can be kept online, and to

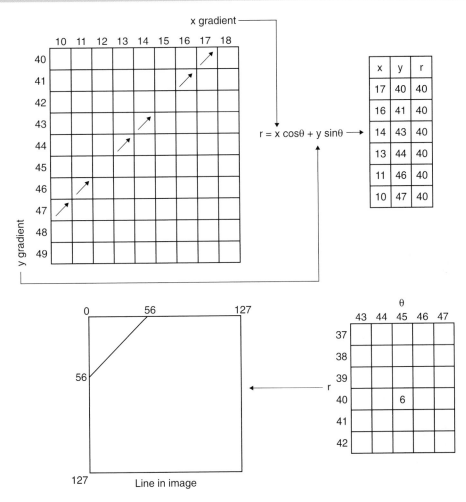

Figure 21 – Hough Transform Process

speed up the subsequent transfer of images either locally or via the internet.

Images are some of the biggest single files that a computer has to deal with, and it is these that many compression programs have been applied to. The over compression of an image was never likely to result in a person's death, however in medical radiology we are dealing with such issues and it must be assured that no compression would result in a patient being misdiagnosed and subsequently receiving an inappropriate course of treatment and subsequently suffering because of this.

This section will first deal with compression as a more general subject, and will then deal with specific compression programs. Finally some of the issues surrounding compression will be discussed more fully.

THE BASICS

There are first some terms that need to be identified and they are summarised in the table 1.

Emerging technology permits ever increasing image resolution, both spatially and in grey level quantisation (the number of grey scales that can be stored), which leads to digital images consisting of large amounts of data. Table 2 shows the varying amounts of memory required for a 35cm × 43cm image with pixel size of 0.1mm in both the x and y directions. This gives a matrix

Table 1 – Basic terminology

Real time compression	Compression takes place with no noticeable delay
Symmetrical compression	Compression and decompression take the same amount of time
Asymmetrical compression	The compression may take a very long time, but subsequent decompression is fast
Lossless compression	There is no loss of image quality between the original and the compressed images
Lossy compression	There is a loss of image quality between the original and the compressed images
Algorithm	Any formula that is applied to an image to compress it

Table 2 – Bit depth, grey levels and file size

Bit Depth	No of grey scales	File Size
8	256	14.35MB
9	512	16.15MB
10	1024	17.94MB
11	2048	19.74MB

of 3500×4300, or a total of 15,050,000 pixels.

The total memory is calculated by multiplying the number of pixels by the bit depth and then dividing by eight. (to convert to bytes) and then dividing by 1 048 576 to convert the bytes to megabytes.

Memory in MB = ((total number of pixels*bit depth)/8)/1048576

Image compression reduces the amount of data needed to represent a digital image. The underlying basis of the reduction process is the removal of redundant data and the aim is to represent an image using a lower number of bits per pixel, without losing the ability to reconstruct the image.

A general algorithm is shown in figure 22.

The first step removes data that is redundant in the image. The second step is to code the transformed data. The image is then stored or transmitted. To retrieve the image the data has to be decoded and then reconstructed.

Data redundancy, R_d in an image can be characterised by the following

$$R_d = 1 - \frac{1}{C_r}$$

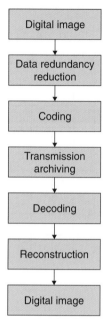

Figure 22 – Compression algorithm

where C_r is called the compression ratio and is given by

$$Cr = \frac{n_1}{n_2}$$

n_1 and n_2 are the number of data in the compressed and uncompressed image. If n_1 and n_2 are equal then the compression ratio is 0 indicating that the original image has no redundant data. If $n_1 \gg n_2$ then C_r tends to infinity and R_d tends towards 1 indicating significant compression and a lot of redundant data.

As an example we will look at one type of data redundancy called interpixel redundancy (see figure 23). We can store this image by scanning line by line and putting the information in the form of a pair of numbers, the first being the value of the grey level of a pixel, then the number of pixels that have the same grey level following it. When the grey level changes a new pair is coded.

As stated previously there are two main techniques of image compression, lossy and lossless. Lossless methods allow the exact reconstruction of all of the individual pixel values whereas lossy does not. One method of loss less compression is via *variable length coding*. We know that each pixel in an image has a grey level represented

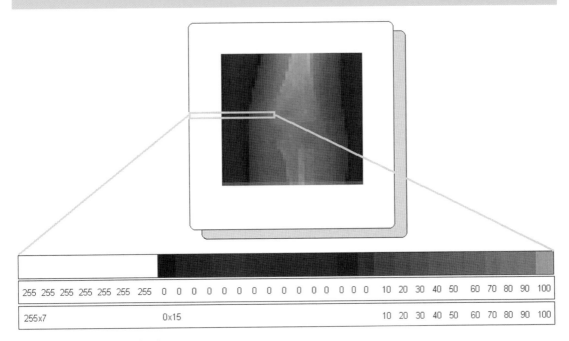

| 255 | 255 | 255 | 255 | 255 | 255 | 255 | 0 | 0 | 0 | 0 | 0 | 0 | 0 | 0 | 0 | 0 | 0 | 0 | 0 | 0 | 0 | 10 | 20 | 30 | 40 | 50 | 60 | 70 | 80 | 90 | 100 |

| 255x7 | 0x15 | 10 | 20 | 30 | 40 | 50 | 60 | 70 | 80 | 90 | 100 |

Figure 23 – Inter pixel redundancy

by an 8 bit code, for example (giving 256 possible levels). Variable length coding essentially takes the most frequently occurring grey levels and assigns them the shortest possible code words.

As an example, take an image that has 8 grey levels. This will take 3 bits to code i.e. $2^3 = 8$.

Table 3 shows the 8 grey levels, the percentage value they occur in the image and the 3 bit code that represents them. The new code is also shown along with the number of bits that are needed.

Table 3 – comparison of binary and decimal

Grey level	Occurrence %	code 1	no. of bits	code 2	no. of bits
g(1)	17	000	3	0	1
g(2)	27	001	3	1	1
g(3)	19	010	3	01	2
g(4)	18	011	3	10	2
g(5)	8	100	3	11	2
g(6)	5	101	3	000	3
g(7)	4	110	3	001	3
g(8)	2	111	3	010	3
	sum = 100		Ave = 3		Ave = 1.49

This is known as Huffman encoding and is utilised in the JPEG algorithm to reduce the amount of information stored.

TRANSFORMATIONS

Fourier transform is a term used frequently in medical imaging and refers to the handling of image data in the frequency domain rather than the spatial domain. From this formula the Discrete Cosine Transform (DCT) has been developed which has several potential uses including compression, filtering and reconstruction. This is the basis of the JPEG (Joint Photographic Expert Group) algorithm and it will be the JPEG algorithm that will be looked at in some detail.

JPEG

JPEG arose from a need to compress 'real world' images to reasonable file sizes. In the 1980s the American National Standards Institute set up a number of working parties to look at the potential for image compression in a number of different fields. A panel of experts reviewed many different algorithms and eventually settled for a standard that is in use today. This was not a truly scientific process but was based more on what they jointly decided looked the best. It is worth bearing in mind that there are several types of JPEG algorithm and new JPEG standards are released periodically. However the basic principles are the same.

Whilst JPEG was set up for the compression of 'real world images' the definition of this can be considered to be an image of constantly changing discrete values, and this is indeed what we have in a digital radiograph. In theory these grey scale images should be equally amenable to compression as their colour counterparts.

As with hardware, the ability of a compression algorithm to stand the test of time depends upon comprehensive standards being laid down initially. JPEG formed ISO standard 10918 and as such is one of the most commonly used formats for images on the internet due to its capabilities to provide good quality images of a small file size.

Small file sizes allow a faster display of a web page and thus user tolerance increases. A further development has been the progressive JPEG where a low-resolution image is displayed first which gradually becomes higher resolution as time allows. This again increases user acceptance as information can be read on the screen whilst the image gradually becomes higher resolution.

Most transformations are capable of achieving compression on certain images but where the DCT is better is that even if in itself it does not achieve high compression ratios it will make the data more amenable to being compressed. It also has the capability of varying the amount of compression that will take place, ranging from lossless (utilising primarily Huffman Encoding) to extremely lossy.

With a grey scale image the first procedure is to break the image up into blocks of 8×8 pixels (figure 24). This is done because the complex mathematics would take up too much processor time if applied to the image as a whole. With recent improvement in processing power 16x16 blocks are now being used, however it is the 8×8 block that will be considered here.

The algorithm then takes the 8×8 image and works out the average pixel value and assigns this to the upper left corner. The deviation from

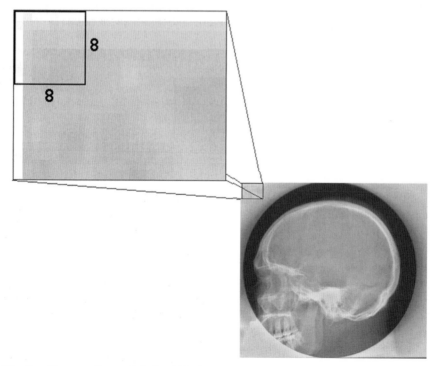

Figure 24 – Breaking up of image into 8×8 blocks

the mean of the other pixel values are then calculated and displayed from the smallest changes
(lowest frequencies) in the upper left, to the
largest changes (highest frequencies) in the
lower right (figure 25).

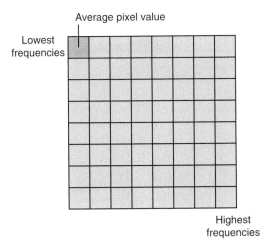

Figure 25 – JPEG ordering of information

The user then selects the level of compression
required. This figure sets the level of a multiplying factor that is more likely to reduce the higher
frequencies to 0. The higher the level of compression chosen the more of the frequencies
that will be set to 0.

When the image is converted back to the spatial domain any pixels with the value 0 are
attributed the average pixel value. The more of

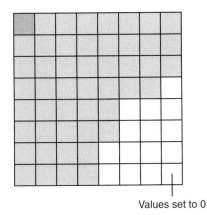

Figure 26 – Low-level compression

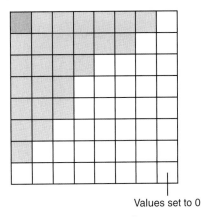

Figure 27 – High-level compression

the pixels that have the same value the larger
the potential within the image for compression.

The effect can be seen utilising histograms. In
figure 28 two levels of compression have been
carried out. As the compression ratio gets larger
the image is broken up into more discrete units,
thus reducing the amount of information that
needs to be encoded.

The first level of compression is quite subtle,
resulting in only a minimal change in the histogram although some degradation of image
quality is already visible.

The second level is quite large and pixelation
(blocking artifact) is clearly visible. The effects on
the histogram are also quite dramatic, resulting
in much less information to store and thus large
compression ratios.

Limitations of JPEG

JPEG is limited in several areas by virtue of the
way it works

Softening Effect

Because the JPEG algorithm removes the higher
frequencies within an image first it has the effect
of softening the edges within an image. Studies
have shown that the human visual system
prefers an image that does not have too many
high frequencies within it and this had lead to
experienced viewers actually preferring images
that have been slightly compressed.

Blocking Artefact

It is because of this segmentation of the image
into 8×8 blocks that excessive compression

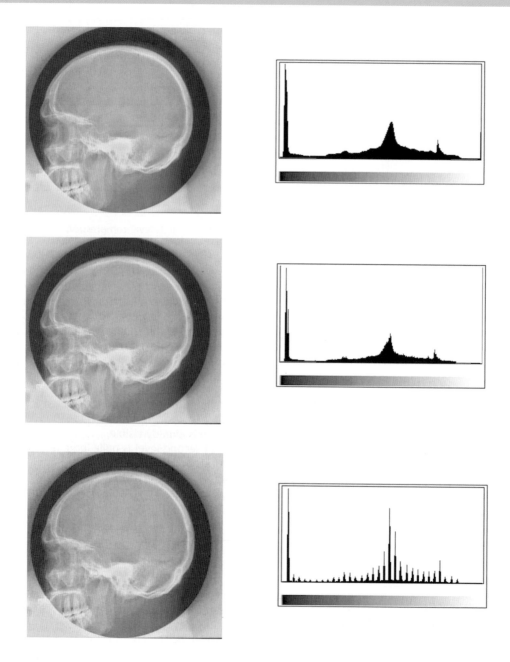

Figure 28 – Effect of levels of compression on histogram

with JPEG can result in what is termed 'blocking artefact'. Any JPEG compression will have this to some extent but it is whether it is discernible that is the important factor. Figure 29 shows the effect of Excessive JPEG compression on an image.

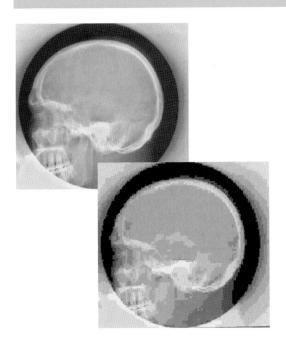

Figure 29 – Excessive JPEG compression of image

Text Compression

JPEG was designed to deal with real world images, and they tend not to have high frequencies within them, such as occur with black text on a white background (such as this page). The result is that any level of compression immediately reduces the sharpness of the text resulting in loss of definition (figure 30). This problem is being addressed for future releases of the JPEG algorithm.

Subsequent Compression

If an image is opened in JPEG format and a change is made to it, such as rotation or addition of text, when it is subsequently saved the compression algorithm is reapplied with a further loss of image detail. This is again being addressed in future editions of JPEG.

REFERENCES AND SOURCES

BOOKS

Carlton R.R., Adler A.M. 1996 **Principles of Radiographic Imaging** Delmar Publishers, London

Carter P.H. 1994 **Chesney's Equipment for Student Radiographers** Blackwell Scientific Publications, London

Davies A., Fennessy P. 1998 **Digital Imaging for Photographers** Focal Press, Oxford

Davies A., Fennessy P. 1994 **Electronic Imaging for Photographers** Focal Press, Oxford

Doi K., Macmahon H., Giger M.L., Hoffman K.R. 1998 **Computer-Aided Diagnosis in Medical Imaging** Elsevier, Amsterdam

Gonzalez R.C., Woods R.E. 1992 **Digital Image Processing** Addison Wesley Publishing Wokingham

Graham R. 1998 **Digital Imaging** Whittles Publishing, Scotland

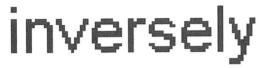

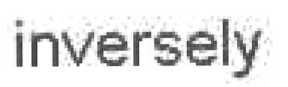

Figure 30– Effects of JPEG compression on text

Greenfield G.B., Hubbard L.B. 1984 **Computers in Radiology** Churchill Livingstone, London

Gunn C. 1994 **Radiographic Imaging** Churchill Livingstone, London

Hajnal J.V., Hill D.L.G., Hawkes D.J. (eds) 2001 **Medical Image Registration** CRC Press, London

Kuni C.C. 1988 **Introduction to Computers and Digital Processing in Medical Imaging** Year Book Medical Publishers, London

Pizzutiello R.J. (ed) 1993 **Introduction to Medical Radiographic Imaging** Eastman Kodak Company, New York

Russ J.C. 1998 **The Image Processing Handbook** CRC Press, London

WWW

http://www.csmc.edu/medphys/MIP.html
Links to image related sites

http://noodle.med.yale.edu/
Image processing analysis group

http://www.jpeg.org
Home of JPEG

9: IMAGE QUALITY AND QUALITY ASSURANCE

Jason Oakley

With special thanks for their invaluable input to:
Anne Davis, Medical Physics Department, Portsmouth Hospitals NHS Trust
Mike Holibinka, Medical Physics Department, Portsmouth Hospitals NHS Trust
Delia Hayes, City University London
Dr Martin Benwell, City University, London
Dr Mic Farquharson, City University, London

This chapter will have to make a careful distinction between the types of modality that exist. Where the subject matter of this chapter refers to all digital images, no matter how they are acquired, the term digital imaging system will be used. Where the text is referring to Indirect or Direct Digital Radiography the term DR will be used. In the same way Computed Radiography will be represented by CR.

INTRODUCTION

Films and intensifying screens have existed relatively unchanged for such a long period that methods of assessing image quality are well established for this technology. All of these methods cannot be applied equally well to the new technologies such as computed and digital radiography. Part One of this chapter will deal with methods of assessing image quality on these modern systems. It aims to give the reader an understanding of what determines quality in a digital image and from this an understanding of how this quality can be assessed.

Quality Assurance (QA) of digital imaging equipment is still a very new area and many developments are being made in assessment methods and tools.

Part Two will look at the tests currently being used to assess individual elements of digital systems and also to assess the system as a whole. Once a method of assessment has been decided upon, it can be implemented simply with a rolling rota of tests. What needs to be taken into account is the potential scale of new tests.

Consider the already demanding number of quality assurance tests currently carried out by both radiographic and medical physics staff. Very few of the x-ray equipment tests will change but eight high quality workstations, 30 medium quality review stations and two hundred standard quality monitors may be added if the system is digital and each will require testing to ensure that optimum quality images are displayed.

There is a very different relationship between exposure and response for film and digital imaging receptors. The response of film follows a sigmoid curve (see grey scale response) and for any exposure the resultant density can be worked out from this curve. Digital imaging systems could be considered as linear in their response, but in reality the response is determined by the parameters set by the user. The response could be adjusted to exactly mimic a current conventional film screen combination or to produce a response that could not be designed into a conventional system.

Because digital imaging systems have such a short history assessment of image quality is particularly important. There are a number of reasons:

- Equipment degradation
  Current quality assurance procedures ensure that conventional equipment is functioning to tolerable standards and the same must be done for the modern technologies. Phosphor storage plates have a finite life, digital radiography cells fail and monitor screens can distort and become damaged by static displays (screen burn – although this is becoming a less of a problem with modern CRT technology).

- Use of Compression
  Any lossey compression technique will result in some loss of image quality, and the magnitude of this effect on the image should be known prior to the compression being implemented on an image. No retrospective correction of image quality is possible with lossey compression techniques unless the raw data is still available. Systems can be designed to choose which images are stored using lossless compression and those which are stored using lossy compression algorithms. Such systems can be considered to be using intelligent archiving.

- Visual Display Units
  The many different types of display monitor are outlined in the equipment section. They range from the standard personal computer monitor to the top of the range reporting workstations. The difference in display quality is enormous, so the quality of image that may appear acceptable on one monitor may not be of diagnostic quality on another, by virtue of the limitations of that monitor.
  If any compression of the image has taken place this will also affect image quality. This may not be a problem on the high quality

workstations, but the effect may be noticeable when added to the limitations of the lower specification monitors. On a low resolution monitor the effect may be amplified to the extent of making the image unusable.

- Printed Images
  When an image is printed there will be some loss of image quality, whatever method is used. In the case of laser printers this comes from converting the digital signal to an analogue waveform to vary the intensity of the laser. In inkjet printers there is a certain amount of spread of ink on the recording media.

- Modality Tolerances
  Each modality will have specific problems that potentially reduce the quality of the image. An example of this would be detector element drop out in a digital radiography plate. During construction several of these will be inadvertently introduced and acceptable levels for grouping, densities and drop out rates will be established by the manufacturer for each modality. Plates that fail this initial test will be rejected. It is the high reject rate during manufacture that keeps the price of flat screen display devices higher than their CRT counterparts.

The above reasons emphasise one of the main problems in assessing digital systems, which is the assessor has to decide which part of the system they are assessing. If you are looking at the quality of the image plate it is hard to do this without looking at the quality of the laser, sampling rate and monitor all at the same time.

It may however be possible to carry out quantitative analysis or visual analysis of image data which excludes the CR / DR viewing station and image printer and this can only be done by transferring image data to Medical Physics for analysis.

This is one reason why any review of digital imaging systems tends to take into account the whole system and not the individual components of the system. This is useful for an overall assessment but does not provide much information about the source of the problem unless the features of the observed artefact are recognisable.

PART ONE: MEASURING IMAGE QUALITY

This section will explore some of the specific parameters that can be measured to indicate image quality. Some of the measurements have their basis in mathematics, to varying degrees of complexity. Where possible the mathematical explanations have been avoided in favour of more practical descriptions. For those who are interested in the formulae behind the final measurements suitable references are given at the end of the chapter.

It is also important to know what part of the system you are assessing. A pre-sampling modulation transfer function or MTF (this section) looks only at the signal coming from the acquisition device. The detected quantum efficiency or DQE (also this section) evaluates the whole system. Using the wrong measure of image quality could result in an over or under estimation of a systems performance.

Another important factor is that if you are using a workstation to assess your image quality there is little point in carrying out any tests until the monitor has been checked and calibrated to operate at optimum levels. What cannot be done as a measure of image quality is to print hard copy film and assess this in the same way that conventional film was assessed. For reasons that will become clear digital film is of a lower resolution than the monitor. These and other factors that will affect image quality will be discussed.

SIMPLE INDICATORS OF IMAGE QUALITY

Spatial Resolution

This can be defined as the smallest difference in distance between two objects that can be distinguished on an imaging system. It is not a measure of how they will actually be perceived by the observer. It may also be different for the separate parts of the imaging system, such as the imaging medium (e.g. the storage plate) the display device (monitor) or the hard copy device (film).

Limiting Resolution (LR)

It is common to describe the spatial resolution capacity of an imaging system in terms of the largest number of line pairs per millimetre (lp/mm) that can be perceived subjectively when an image of a resolution grating (line pair test tool) is produced.

Such a test should not really be necessary for digital radiography systems because the limiting resolution will be determined by the pixel size. Pixel size depends on the image field size relative to the image matrix size and two pixels will be required to demonstrate one line pair. However the pixel size represents the limiting resolution of the system and the actual resolution of a digital imaging system may be below this

Hence, for example, an 18 × 24 cm plate in a CR system with a 1770 × 2370 matrix (the rate at which it is being sampled) will result in a limiting resolution of 5 line pairs per mm.

(180mm/1770 = 0.1mm horizontal resolution, so for a high contrast object the smallest change in frequency that can be recorded will be in 0.2 mm. This gives a limiting resolution in the horizontal direction of 5 lp/mm.)

The image of a line pair test tool could not yield a better result in this case so the limiting resolution for a digital system is the same as the Nyquist limit (see next).

In a direct digital system the individual charge coupled devices (CCDs) that will store the information will have a finite 'dead space' between them so the number of CCDs does not determine the resolution. Instead the resolution is taken as the space from the middle of one CCD to the centre of the next (figure 1).

Pixel size

The pixel size in the x direction = length of image field in x direction/no of pixels in x direction.

The pixel size in the y direction = length of image field in y direction/no of pixels in y direction.

Two directions are considered because the

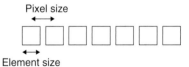

Pixel size

Element size

Figure 1 – CCD resolution

pixels may not be square. MRI is an example where the pixels are often rectangular. With CR devices it is also common for the resolution to be higher in the x plane (the fast scan direction) as the CR plate is scanned linearly and then a slight decrease in resolution in the y plane as the laser moves down to scan the next row in the x plane (slow scan direction).

So whilst a matrix size of 512 × 512 offers the potential for greater resolution than a 256 × 256 matrix it is impossible to tell without knowing the size of the imaged area. For example if a 512 × 512 matrix were applied to an imaged area 50mm × 50mm the size of each pixel would be 0.1 × 0.1mm (equivalent to 5 line pairs per mm (lp/mm) − see limiting resolution). If a 256 × 256 matrix were applied to an image 20mm × 20mm, the size of each pixel would be 0.08 × 0.08 mm (in excess of 6 lp/mm).

The pixel size is only a very basic measurement of the resolution capability of the system but it does however give an indication of the potential limiting resolution of the final image. Actual resolution is also influenced by the cross-sectional area of the scanning laser or spot size (i.e. stimulation of adjacent areas of detector when collection is not taking place so degrading signal) and scatter of laser light within the phosphor (See Chapter Three − Equipment).

In the same way knowing the matrix size of an image is not enough to make an evaluation of the spatial resolution. In addition to this it is necessary to know either the size of the imaged field or the size of the field of view (FOV).

In a similar way it is important to know the thickness of a voxel (a pixel that also has depth − See Chapter 2 − Basics) with in tomographic or volume acquisition technologies. The spatial resolution in the x,y axis is not limited by length in the z axis (thickness of the voxel) provided the test detail spans the full length of the voxel and is correctly aligned. In CT, larger voxels are subject to partial volume effects that affect contrast and noise levels as the larger the voxel the greater the number of photons absorbed. In planar systems the only information that is being obtained is x,y, so the thicker the detector element the great the quantum conversion efficiency up to the limit where the element thickness inhibits signal collection. There is also greater possibility of light spread to adjacent elements or for oblique photons having the same original causing signal generation in adjoining elements.

For cross sectional imaging modalities the thinner the voxel the more accurate the final representation will be of the signal from that area but, because less signal has gone to make up the final pixel that is seen, the signal to noise ratio will be reduced. Increasing the exposure and thus restoring the signal to noise ratio but keeping the accurate pixel value, can counter this. This will, of course, increase the dose to the patient. As in many aspects of medical imaging there is a balance between image quality and patient exposure to be sought. Trade-offs are made until an acceptable balance is identified.

Nyquist limit

Nyquist theorem states that if you have frequency of f, then in order to sample this frequency correctly the sampling frequency must be at least 2f. For example if you wish to have the equivalent resolution of 5 lp/mm then each line pair will be 0.2mm. To sample this correctly the sampling rate must be at least 0.1mm, or double the frequency that we wish to see.

If the sampling rate is too coarse or the system is not capable of resolving such detail then an artefact can appear known as aliasing.

In CR this is determined by the sampling rate (speed of laser and digitisation frequency) of the laser and thus the pixel size depends upon the laser scan.

Other factors affecting the limiting resolution of a CR system are;

- Size of laser spot
- Scattering of laser light (in exactly the same way as light scatters within a fluorescent screen in a conventional cassette)
- Scattering of photo stimulated light (again similar to conventional screens)

In DR the limiting resolution is determined by the size of the sensors and the distance between the sensors in the flat panel detector (figure 2).

However, because of the arrangement of the detectors there is always the possibility that the stated resolution may not always be accurate. (figure 2)

Here the test tool has the same theoretical spatial resolution as the detector. However theorem states that to sample an image accurately you have to sample at twice the highest frequency of that image (the Nyquist frequency) and this is not possible in this scenario.

The correct sampling of detail is an important factor in digital imaging according to the features of anatomy being imaged.

With conventional film screen combinations the resolution in the x and y directions (and any combinations of these) is comparable because of the even distribution of approximately equally sized grains of silver within the film emulsion. This is not always the case with computed radiography and digital radiography acquisition devices because whilst the plates will have a similar construction to film the plates are read in such a way that the resolutions differs in the x and y directions (fast and slow scan directions).

There is also a potential problem with the way in which the test tool is orientated. Figure 3 shows the magnified effect of rotating a lp/mm test tool within a matrix, and the loss of definition of the borders. With a CR plate this affect may be enhanced due to the reduction in measured resolution in the fast-scan and slow-scan directions, which may not be equal, whilst the detector's resolution (the CR plate) is uniform. This affect does not require such a large rotation to be seen. If a test tool is only slightly misaligned with the pixels the affect will be seen.

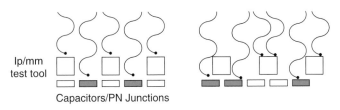

lp/mm test tool

Capacitors/PN Junctions

Figure 2 – Problems associated with test tool alignment

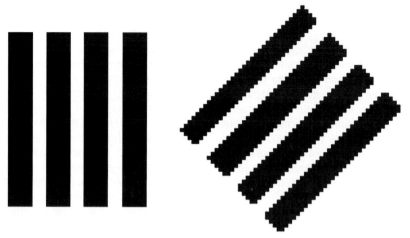

Figure 3 – Effect of rotation on image resolution

Contrast and Brightness

The next two sections will look at the effect of contrast on brightness on the appearance of an image. It will be re-iterated several times that once a monitor has been set up using a test tool (such as the SMPTE) to optimum brightness and contrast levels for the viewing conditions that it should not be altered. This level will vary from monitor to monitor depending upon viewing conditions, ambient lightning, reflections etc. Autos sensing systems are available that ensure optimum viewing conditions in areas affected by varying light levels

The brightness and contrast alterations should then be done using the software (window width, window level and look up tables) and not the monitor adjustment.

Effects of Contrast

The amount of inherent contrast in an image is a very important parameter of image quality. Any x-ray imaging device must be capable of representing contrast between structures with different attenuation co-efficients, and the ability of a system to do this is demonstrated by how well these structures can be distinguished from one another on the final image. This is known as contrast sensitivity.

As long as the imaging system is capable of recording this contrast the software should allow the image to be manipulated to demonstrate it.

Adjusting the visual contrast (this is distinct from acquired contrast which is determined by the kV, primary signal read and processing) may produce a very black and white image if the contrast is high, or a very grey image if the contrast is low (see figure 4). This is manipulated by windowing and levelling or may be pre-determined according to image read/display protocols defined within the CR/DR display system.

The amount of contrast in an image is very important when considering the effect of noise on an image. The ability to discriminate structures with subtle differences in contrast is affected by the noise in the image. Detected quantum efficiency (DQE) –which is discussed later in this section, takes other factors into account and therefore assesses the system as a whole.

Effects of Brightness

Brightness is a user-defined parameter but is also relative to external factors such as ambient light levels. It can, however, have an effect on image quality, especially if the final images are being printed onto hard copy and this is the only image that the end users will see. This is one of the justifications for all digital images being viewed on a computer that allows software manipulation of brightness (and contrast) values.

There should be no need for the users to adjust the monitor once it has been set to optimum levels. Figure 5 shows the effects of bright-

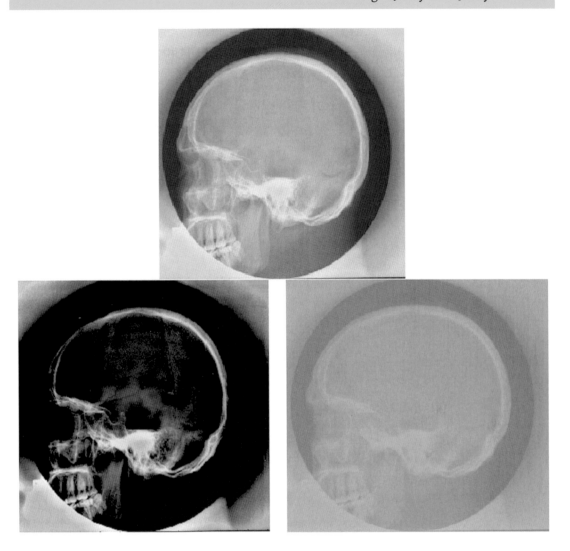

Figure 4 – Effects of normal, high and low contrast on image quality

ness adjustment on image quality utilising software.

Adjusting the brightness of the monitor would have a similar effect on image quality, and more importantly mean that any subsequent software driven manipulations would be displayed inaccurately.

Luminosity

Luminosity is a measure of brightness of the wavelengths of light that are emitted from an object. It may be possible to adjust the luminosity of the monitors chosen for your system. Often the engineer makes this adjustment on installation. Whatever the case it is important

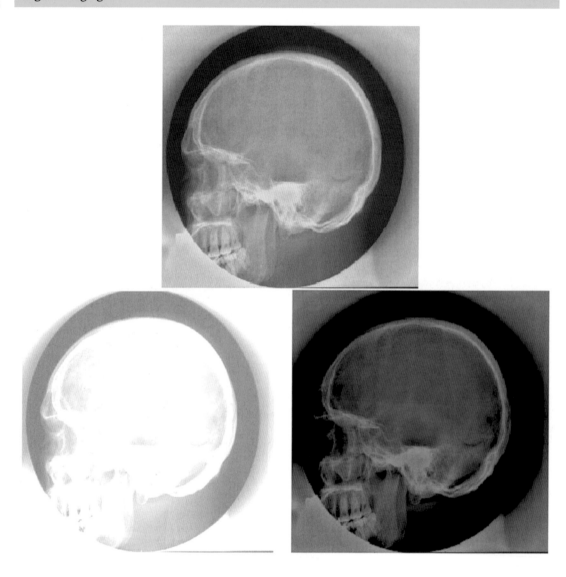

Figure 5 – Effects of normal, high and low brightness on image quality

that all monitors are as similar as possible in luminosity on installation.

Luminosity can be calibrated using a photometer and white test image that can be recorded and used as a bench mark against which regular testing can be performed. It should be remembered that luminosity will vary greatly between monitors of different quality and also between colour and black and white monitors. Monitors should be calibrated to be the same as other monitors of the same type and not against different classes of monitors.

Grey Scale Response

The grey scale response of conventional x-ray film is primarily down to the sensitometric curve for each film screen combination. In digital radiography the response is governed by parameters programmed by the user (which may be preset) and determine the appearance of the final image (see figure 6). These are generally set to achieve optimum image quality for each examination. On graphs the relationship is often drawn as linear, but the graph may take any form, depending on the parameters set.

Dynamic Range

This is the ability of the system to record varying intensities of photons. A wide dynamic range is important if the low photon flux through highly attenuating parts of the anatomy and the high photon flux around image boundaries or through structures that hardly attenuate the beam at all are all to be detected. Detectors can also be swamped with signal that can corrupt the image data or result in artefacts. This is different to energy sensitivity, which can be understood by looking at quantum conversion efficiency at different energies, i.e. the energy efficiency curve.

Some systems may not record very low energy photons, and thus an exposure made up of a low photon flux will give a very poor image, and conversely another may not be able to record high levels of photon energy. Both of these extremes will have implications for patient dose.

The ideal system will be able to make use of all of the varying energies within the beam incident upon the transducer to produce the final image.

Noise

Noise is an unwanted disturbance in an otherwise useful signal. It has the effect of reducing image quality. Noise in any imaging system can detract from the useful information and reduce the contrast resolution perceptible in the images produced. Noise can come from many sources including:

- Quantum noise – interactions between x-ray photons and the phosphor screen. Due to statistical variations in the photon flux, which depends on the intensity of the beam, and subsequent efficiency of the recording medium, photo-multiplier tubes etc
- Electronic noise – photo multiplier tubes (PMTs), amplifiers, detectors etc.
- Structural noise – pattern of crystals etc (no structural noise with amorphous selenium due to the columnar structure of crystals)
- Digitisation noise – if the image display is operating at 256 grey levels and the imaging acquisition device is acquiring 1024 discrete levels, every four-acquisition levels will be merged into one grey scale. Most systems run on 10 bit (1024 grey scales) to avoid this. However new systems are arriving that will utilise 14,15 and even 16 bits.

(The viewing monitor can introduce further noise as can the film and processing when hard copies are taken of the acquired images.)

The overall amount of noise in a system is

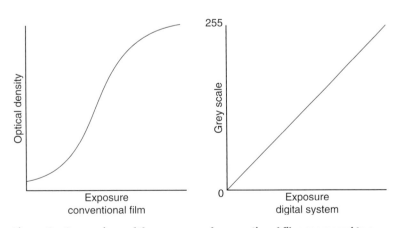

Figure 6 – Comparison of the response of conventional film compared to a digital imaging system

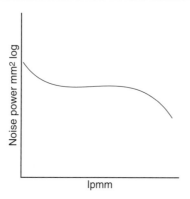

Figure 7 – Noise power spectrum

known as its power and it may be made of low frequencies (coarse) or high frequencies (fine). The power of noise is its amplitude squared.

To describe the noise characteristics of an imaging system, a noise power spectrum (or Wiener spectrum) is often produced and presented as a graph of the amount or power of the noise against the spatial frequency at which it occurs. Very fine fluctuations of density arising from phosphor storage grain size, for example, would be seen at the high frequency end of the spectrum whereas quantum noise would tend to be altogether coarser and would be seen at the lower spatial frequencies.

The noise power spectrum can also be use to compare systems, and will highlight frequencies at which the digital imaging system is less efficient and explanations of this inefficiency can then be sought.

The response of the imaging system to a uniform, overall exposure should be to produce, over the whole image field, a value of density, brightness or pixel value that is the same in each area. Noise will cause the values to differ across the field and these variations are essentially what is meant by the term noise.

In a noise power spectrum the noise is defined as exposure fluctuations rather than variations in optical density, brightness or pixel values. In a digital system, the exposure values would be obtained from the pixel values by relating them to the appropriate transfer or gamma curve.

The noise present in the image from any system can be expected to vary with the level of radiation exposure used to produce the image. If more quanta are incident then the difference

between the noise and useful image becomes larger. The converse is that the exposure to the patient is increased. This effect can be seen in CT where if too little exposure is given the image appears very grainy. If more exposure is given then the image looks crisper due to the increased signal to noise ratio.

Figure 8 looks at the effects of increased noise on image quality for a low contrast object.

The first image in figure 8 shows an image devoid of any noise. The histogram shows only two levels of grey meaning that the signal to noise ratio is high. As the noise becomes progressively worse the signal to noise ratio is reduced. As the noise increases the amplitude of the peaks decreases (large numbers of these pixels are being altered in value by noise). Resulting in a spread of each of the peaks. As the noise increases further the histogram shows a typical spread around the mean pixel value for the image with both of the peaks eventually being lost in the noise. Characteristic noise peaks at both the white and black ends of the histogram can also be seen.

The visibility of objects being imaged can be affected by the amount of noise in an image. Small objects of low contrast are most affected as the signal from these details is more closely matched to the properties of the noise. The effect is less marked if the contrast difference, or subject contrast, is high. Figure 9 shows the effects of increasing noise on small details of both high and low contrast. The high contrast images maintain a higher signal to noise, compared to the low contrast images where the noise amplitude becomes comparable with the signal amplitude.

High contrast images typically tolerate noise better than the low contrast images and it is for this reason that detective quantum efficiency (DQE) takes into account both of these factors when assessing the overall quality of a system.

DQE is related to SNR^2 and noise equivalent quanta (NEQ). NEQ is dependent upon the modulation transfer function (MTF), Noise Power Spectrum (NPS), and Large Area Signal LAS (average pixel value in an image). The spatial frequency response and the noise level at different spatial frequencies also affect DQE. It is perhaps worthwhile mentioning that DQE is by no means simple to measure.

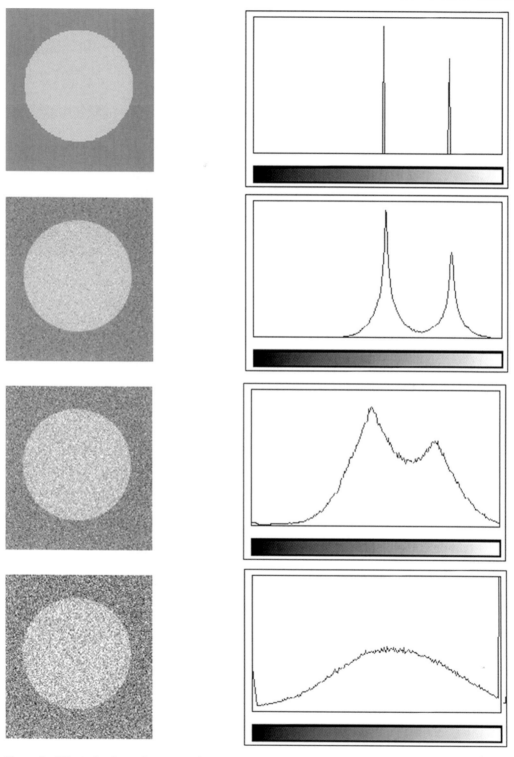

Figure 8 – Effect of noise on image quality

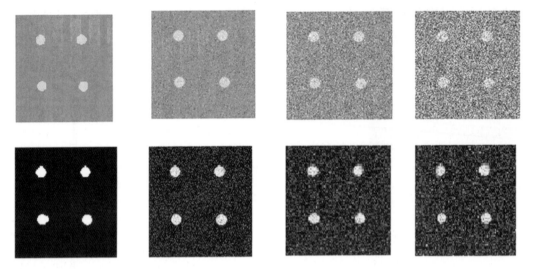

Figure 9 – Low contrast and high contrast images degraded by noise

Measurement of Quality

Whilst the above parameters affect image quality, they are not indicators of the actual level of quality. The following sections deal with measurements that could be considered figures of merit that allow systems to be compared.

Large Area Signal

This is the average pixel value in an image and can be worked out in many most image software packages.

Pre-sampling MTF

The modulation transfer function (MTF) describes the ability of a system to record the spatial frequencies that are available to be recorded

$$MTF = \frac{output\ modulation}{input\ modulation}$$

The MTF is the ratio of the spatial frequencies of the image over the spatial frequencies of the input object. A perfect imaging system would have an MTF of 1.0 at all spatial frequencies, thus representing the image perfectly.

The radiation pattern incident on the recording medium may be thought of, for example, as the input amplitude and in the case of a lp/mm test tool would take the form of a square wave. The corresponding density or brightness levels in the final image would be the output ampli-

tude. If the output amplitude were exactly the same as the input amplitude it would also be a square wave. The closer the ratio is to 1.0 (or to 100%) the better the MTF of the system. As the MTF decreases the wave will get further from being a 100% of the amplitude towards being a flat line with 0% modulation (see figure 10).

The MTF is known as the pre-sampled MTF because it is taken prior to the sampling of the waveform and thus it is prior to digitisation.

The MTF is likely to be very good for low frequency input amplitude signals (low resolution), which will be slowly changing or well spaced but will fall off as the detail to be imaged becomes finer (higher spatial frequencies). The common way of displaying a MTF of a system is as a graph with MTF on the vertical axis and spatial frequency (in line pairs per mm) on the horizontal axis. (See Figure 12.)

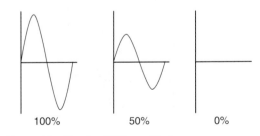

Figure 10 – Varying MTF amplitudes

At lower spatial frequencies the MTF is likely to be high (towards 1.0), meaning that the changes in density would be clearly visible on the image. As the line pairs get closer together less quanta will be recorded and thus conversion from the actual line pairs to the digital image will be less (towards 0), meaning that the smaller spatial frequencies will be more difficult if not impossible to see.

The highest spatial frequency visible tends to be at an MTF of about 4% and corresponds to the limiting resolution determined subjectively by viewing the image of a line pair test tool. At this point the signal is only 4% of the input modulation and may only be just visible. (When considering the MTFs of different imaging systems, it is common to compare the spatial frequencies at which the MTFs are 50%.)

MTF can be can also be explained as the Fourier Transform of the line spread function (LSF) of a system and in a conventional radiographic system the line spread function is derived from the image of a 10-micron slit in a tungsten test tool.

For the MTF to be derived from a LSF the response must be isotropic i.e. it is the same in all directions (unless the direction in which the LSF and hence MTF are derived is stated from which the MTF can be correctly interpreted). This may not be true for digital images so it is important that the MTF is given parallel and perpendicular to the scanning direction.

With digital images (where the analogue imaging signal is sampled and digitised) the Fourier Transform can again present the problem of aliasing if under sampling of the image input signal has occurred. The rate of sampling has to be at least twice the rate at which the signal is changing if it is to be represented correctly (Nyquist theorem). Essentially, this means that if the analogue signal contained information at higher spatial frequencies than the system's Nyquist limit those higher spatial frequencies could not be shown in the digital image − and in the discrete Fourier Transform they could be aliased i.e. represented inaccurately as lower frequencies than they really are. Figure 11 should be comprised of very fine vertical lines but due to the lines being finer than the limiting resolution of the system they have been aliased to lower frequencies. In this case it has produced diagonal lines across the image.

This potential problem of aliasing would make the MTF inaccurate − so for digital imaging systems it is pre- sampling MTFs which are compared. Hence it is the imaging capability of the analogue components of the system that is described rather than the whole system. This is important to bear in mind when comparing imaging systems.

It is possible for the MTF for each part of the imaging chain to be calculated and this can be used to give the MTF for the whole system, which will always be lower than the pre-sampled MTF. The DQE can be used to give an overall value which takes into account the MTF, Noise

Fig 11 − Aliasing due to under sampling or exceeding the limiting resolution of a system

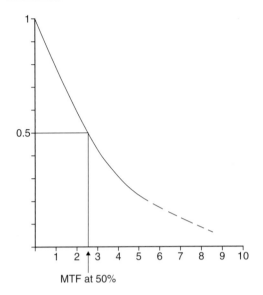

MTF at 50%

Figure 12 – Example of MTF curve

Table 1 – Examples of NEB for Fuji CR system

	NEBs in cycles per mm	
	Horizontal	Vertical
18×24ST	2.31	2.31
18×24HR	3.35	3.4
35×43ST	1.91	2.23

For the high-resolution plate, the figures are 6 line pairs, 2.2 line pairs and 3.35 cycles per mm respectively. *(MDD Evaluation Report MDD/92/36)*. The higher the NEB the higher the resolution.

LR, MTF and NEB describe the spatial resolution characteristics of a system and may all be used to define its limitations.

Power spectrum and dose efficiency of the system i.e. which evaluates the whole digital imaging system.

The relationships of these factors can be shown using the following formulas:

$$NEQ = MTF^2/(NPS/LAS^2)$$
$$DQE = NEQ/Q$$

(where Q is the number of photons).

Noise Equivalent Bandwidth (NEB)

NEB is now considered one of the most accurate figures for allowing a quick comparison of the limiting resolution of different systems, and is also a good indicator of how sharp the final image will appear. The figure is worked out from twice the integral of the MTF^2 value at each spatial frequency between zero and the Nyquist limit for the system. It is again important for the NEB to be quoted in both the scan direction and perpendicular to it (table 1).

The NEB is more appropriate than the MTF for comparing digital systems, but quite often a number of different parameters are given that will allow comparisons of the ability of digital imaging systems.

E.g. the limiting resolution for a standard Fuji 18×24cm imaging plate is 5 line pairs per mm; the 50% MTF is 1.5 line pairs per mm and the NEB is 2.31 cycles per mm.

Noise Equivalent Quanta (NEQ)

If the MTF of a system at a particular frequency MTF(f) expresses how well the image represents information at that frequency in the subject (the real signal), the relationship between the MTF(f) and the noise power at the same frequency may be thought of as an indication of the signal to noise ratio of a system. The MTF is a figure of the signal possible at spatial frequencies and the noise power spectrum (NPS) is the amount of noise at these spatial frequencies. The square of this signal to noise ratio is known as the Noise Equivalent Quanta (NEQ) of a system.

A certain amount of x-ray quanta are incident on the detecting medium per unit area (the signal) to produce an image. These x-ray quanta may not all be detected and their input may be degraded by noise processes. The NEQ is intended to indicate the flux density of x-ray quanta that are actually used to produce the resultant image as opposed to the density of quanta incident on the detector.

It is often described as the amount of exposure that would have been required if the imaging system were 100% perfect, and all of the quanta within the x-ray beam were used. The higher the NEQ the higher the SNR.

Detective Quantum Efficiency (DQE)

It should be noted that DQE is not the same as the quantum detection efficiency (QDE) of intensifying screens.

In the ideal imaging system 100% of the x-ray quanta that reach the recording media (CR or DR plate) would be used to create the image. DQE is the relationship between the density of useful quanta (the NEQ) and the density of x-ray quanta actually incident on the detector:

$$DQE = \frac{NEQ}{Q}$$

Where Q is the actual quanta incident on the digital imaging system. So the best DQE value for a system would be 1.0 or 100%, indicating that in this instance all of the quanta produced are used to make up the image and that no noise goes to make up any of the signal within the image. This of course, is not the case in real imaging systems.

The signal that we get out of the system will not be entirely made up from just the signal generated by the quanta. The signal will also, to varying degrees, be made up of noise. If our signal is 80% of the quanta incident upon the detection device we cannot assume that the device is 80% efficient because an allowance must be made for the noise within the image, thus reducing this figure. Other factors such as the amount of contrast in the image are also taken into account when calculating the DQE as a high contrast image will be less effected by noise.

The DQE, by taking these other variables into account is demonstrated on a graph very much like the MTF curves, but evaluating the whole system. Where as the MTF curve is a pre-sampling measurement, and is often measured in ideal conditions, the DQE is a measurement of the real performance of a system at the end stage. It is because of this that it is currently being used along with limiting resolution and the NEB to define the overall performance of a system.

CR/DR Artefacts
Now that several methods of measuring image quality have been identified it is important to look at other variables that may affect image quality. In the same way as conventional film screen combinations may be effected by artefacts there are several artefacts that are peculiar to digital imaging systems.

An artefact can be considered to be anything that appears on the image that is not part of what would constitute the perfect image. This section will briefly outline each artefact and where appropriate suggest ways of suppressing or removing them

Quantum Mottle
Whilst not being a true artefact quantum mottle can have a large effect on image quality. In the early days of computed radiography (CR) there was a misconception that large dose reduction would be possible and accordingly exposures were considerably reduced. The software will attempt to optimise how the image is displayed. However if the underexposed image is looked at closely, a lack of detail is evident.

It is important when any new imaging system is installed that the exposure factors used match the imaging system to give the best quality image for the lowest dose possible (ALARP – as low as reasonably practicable). The Medical Physics Department should be called on to help in the initial setting of exposure factors and these should be clearly displayed on exposure charts.

Screen marks
These are caused by dirt on the surface of the phosphor plates or by scratches within the protective surface. Routine cleaning will help to ensure that their appearance is kept to a minimum.

Printer Artefacts
These most commonly appear as horizontal or vertical lines that have failed to print. Other artefacts that can appear are bands of increased density where the film has not moved through the printer at an even rate. Some can be rectified by running the printer's own diagnostic program, but others will require the replacement of components such as the thermal head, and will necessitate the services of an engineer.

Film Artefacts
Film will record any image faults originating in other parts of the system, but can also introduce artefacts of its own. It is possible, for example for the films to be damaged. 'Laser' film, as it is often called is prone to damage by direct heat, and can also be scratched.

Element Failure
In most flat panels it is extremely likely that several of the elements will have failed during man-

ufacture, and software compensation will have been incorporated. The software may not automatically compensate for subsequent element failures however, and in this case areas of failure may become visible.

Background Noise

Phosphor storage plates are very sensitive to scattered radiation and if the cassette is not used frequently scatter can be visible on the image as background noise. Imaging plates must be erased regularly.

Saturation

Even a computed radiography or digital system has a limit to its dynamic range. Once this is exceeded saturation has occurred and no more quanta can be stored. This can result in areas of maximum density (black) on the image, that even when manipulated using software do not reveal any detail within them. If this happens to the whole image then the system may refuse to read the plate as no image will be discernible and the plate will have to be erased.

Part one of this section has outlined the various elements that go to make up image quality, and the measurements that can be made to objectively assess the quality of the image. Part Two will now look at how image quality can be assessed on an ongoing basis.

PART TWO: QUALITY ASSURANCE TESTS

Any tests that are carried out need to be reproducible and generate data that can be compared on an ongoing basis to detect varying image quality. They also need to be realistic for the team of people expected to carry them out. For this reason this section will be divided into simple and complex system testing.

SIMPLE QUALITY ASSURANCE TESTS

Any digital system evaluation should start with ensuring that the monitor settings are optimal before continuing to test the performance of digital imaging system.

MONITOR TESTS

Grey scale display

One of the main issues with display screen equipment is the capability to display grey levels (especially on colour monitors). It is very easy to adjust your PC monitor to alter the way the image looks. You can experiment with this by altering the greyscale for yourself with any image on the screen, but be careful to make a note of the original settings. Figure 13 shows the effects of altering the brightness and contrast of an image.

It is clear that only A shows the full grey scale and that each of the others removes some part of the information that it is possible to see. If the monitor is set so that all the grey scales are visible then any image that is displayed subsequently has the potential to be seen in its entirety. If the user then manipulates the image using the software then the image may be altered in a meaningful way . If the user then wishes to revert to the original image this can be done at the click

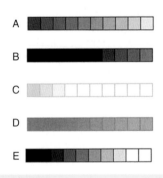

A – The original grey scale
B – Brightness reduced
C – Brightness increased
D – Contrast reduced
E – Contrast increased

Figure 13 – Effects of altering brightness and contrast on a simple grey scale

of a mouse button, as the brightness and contrast of the monitor are still the same.

A standard grey scale needs to be decided upon for all monitors to be calibrated to. This will ensure that each monitor will display any image to its best ability, and will take into account some other factors such as the level of ambient lighting (if the test is done in less than perfect viewing conditions). Many grey scale test images are kept to below twenty discrete steps between 0 and 255 grey levels. This is because of the limitations of the human visual system when looking at grey scale images.

The grey scale test is a test that will need to be carried out frequently to ensure that the monitors have not been altered by the users. Alternatively the test grey scale can be incorporated into an opening screen which requests that the users check the grey scale before moving on to review images.

Geometric Distortion

Monitors now come with a variety of geometric distortion tools that are normally accessed in the same way as the brightness and contrast. Common distortions are shown in figure 14.

It is not always apparent when slight distortion has occurred and it is therefore necessary to ensure that distortion tests are a part of the quality assurance programme. Most monitors come with software built in that allows manual correction of distortion

Degaussing

Degaussing is used to demagnetise the metal shadow mask (see Equipment − Monitors) if it becomes magnetised by external forces such as the Earth's magnetic field or nearby audio devices. This can lead to the monitor's electron beam being deflected and producing a distorted image. Most monitors now come with a utility to degauss that can be run by the user.

It should also become common practice that the brightness and contrast controls on monitors should not be adjusted to change images once they have been optimally set. Only the image display software should be used to adjust image quality.

Other than simple 'user' evaluation of the monitor there are several more robust tests that have been devised. The need for them arose from the development of image intensifiers and subsequently the transmission of the fluoroscopy image to a television monitor as opposed to a direct viewing of a phosphor plate. The display of the image using an electronic device (the monitor) became

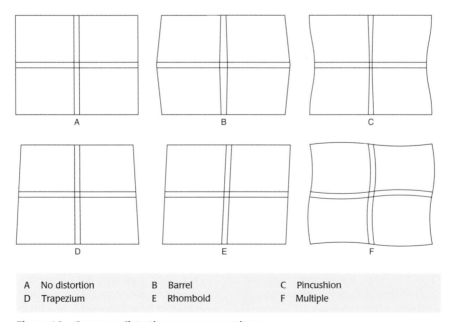

| A | No distortion | B | Barrel | C | Pincushion |
| D | Trapezium | E | Rhomboid | F | Multiple |

Figure 14 − Common distortions seen on monitors

an important part of the imaging chain

Readers familiar with diagnostic imaging departments may know some of the Leeds test objects produce by Faxil, which can be used to test the image acquisition and subsequent display.

Any tests undertaken with these test tools will evaluate the system as a whole and will not take into account the monitor alone. For this reason software programs have been developed to allow assessment of the monitor without acquiring an image first. Thus variables introduced by the imaging system will not affect the result.

An example of this is the SMPTE test tool that is used to check for image distortion, grey scale reproduction, limiting resolution (at both high and low contrast) and uniformity. Other programs allow a more thorough evaluation of colour monitors.

Cassette and Imaging Plate (Storage Plate) Checks

CR cassettes should be checked for damage on a regular basis, and faulty cassettes removed from service or repaired. The light tight requirements of conventional cassettes no longer apply as CR cassettes can stand a long period of exposure to daylight, but a good seal is still important to protect the phosphor plate inside from fluids.

The imaging plates undergo a lot of travel in their lifetime, being constantly removed from the cassette to be read and then replaced. A regular check of imaging plates should be made for scratches that could affect image quality. Subsequent testing of the plates must be undertaken if scratches are found. It may be possible to remove some marks when cleaning the cassettes, but if the marks persist then the plate should be removed from service.

Most plates have an estimated life of 10,000 exposures. It is possible in some systems for the plates to fall from the cassettes, if they are inadvertently opened. This physical damage may well shorten their life and all plates should be inspected and cleaned following such incidents.

The plates are also sensitive to scatter radiation and over time, to light. This means that if a cassette is not used for a substantial period it can become 'fogged'. Any subsequent image acquired will be visible but will be built upon a layer of background noise. This can be avoided by regularly 'erasing' all of the cassettes at the

start of every day. Exposure of the imaging plate to a row of very bright fluorescent lights within the reader will result in the removal of any electrons still trapped within the phosphor. Some systems incorporate this function into the reading process and it is performed automatically after each exposed plate has been scanned.

Digital Radiography (DR) panels are more delicate by virtue of the complex electronics that they contain and the panels and their cables should be inspected very carefully for damage. A simple test for uniformity viewed at maximum magnification can be used to check for failed elements that will be seen as areas of no signal in the otherwise uniform field.

Printer Checks

Most printers provide a test image that can be printed out to check the printer quality at any given time. Many faults will first become apparent during day-to-day printing, but if the error occurs gradually it may not be noticeable until it becomes serious. Periodic testing of the system is therefore very important.

In addition all of the tests that are carried out on the monitor (LR, TCDD, grey scale, uniformity etc) should be performed to check that the printed image reproduces the monitor image as closely as possible. There will always be some degradation of the image quality when using any form of printer.

It is interesting to compare the QA test carried out using the monitor to the test carried out using the hardcopy film. The results can show a surprising amount of image quality reduction between the two devices.

Threshold Contrast Detail Detectability (TCDD)

This test can be used to evaluate the image quality of the monitor, and if the images are hard copied the printer and film as well. There are many test objects available to carry this out, such as the Leeds Test Objects (TO10, TO12, TO16, TO20). A comparison of the results yielded from these two can enhance the users understanding of the differences in viewing images on a monitor and on a hard copy medium such as film.

For radiographers an understanding of the parameters discussed so far may be useful in reviewing literature about new imaging systems and comparing their imaging properties. It is, however, precise and time consuming work to produce MTFs or noise power spectra and an x-ray department is unlikely to undertake these assessments for itself because there is unlikely to be the time or the equipment available to do so.

The overall performance of an imaging system may be assessed subjectively, however, with the use of a threshold contrast detail detectability (TCDD) test object. Faxil in Leeds produces such objects and they are calibrated for use at specific kVps with specific levels of copper filtration of the x-ray beam. From the outside they look like large black plastic discs. Inside they contain details to be imaged. The TO. 16-test tool has details in twelve different sizes (11.1mm to 0.25 mm diameters) and each different size has details of twelve different x-ray attenuation coefficients that will produce twelve different contrasts when exposed under the correct exposure conditions.

The resulting images can be printed onto film and viewed under optimum and consistent viewing conditions (light boxes for example can vary tremendously in performance) by a group of experienced observers. The observers look at each group of details and record the number of details seen in each group. This permits the threshold contrast (TC) to be determined for each detail size.

In general, the higher the value of the threshold index the better the system is at visualising contrast and detail. This is a test which could easily be incorporated into a departments quality assurance procedures for its digital imaging systems.

Uniformity

Test tools are available or a plate can simply be exposed through filtration of 1.5mm Cu. The resultant image can be looked at for obvious areas of increased or decreased density, but a more practical method is to reduce the matrix size of the image to 30 × 30 pixels. This will average a number of pixels together and make any non-uniformity more obvious.

Figure 15 shows first the original image acquired at full resolution. The image was they reduced in size to 30 × 40 pixels and the contrast of the image altered to enhance any difference in the uniformity of the image. The dark band running horizontally across the image should be a cause for concern.

Resolution

A simple check can be carried out using a resolution test tool but bear in mind that there will be a Nyquist limit for the system and the imaging device will not be able to display details beyond this. The maximum number of line pairs distinguished by a number of observers can be assessed on installation and the same test repeated at regular intervals. It is important to standardise viewing conditions and the level of compression that an image has undergone.

It should be borne in mind that like the TCDD this is a subjective test and is operator and exposure dependent. However it can be of interest to compare the manufacturers claims of limiting resolution to the actual perceived resolution that must be equal to or less than the Nyquist limit of

Figure 15 – Uniformity test

the system. Howeer it must be borne in mind that the manufacturers will have acquired their data under laboratory conditions and so matching exactly what was done previously is very complex matter.

SYSTEM QUALITY ASSURANCE (COMPLEX)

Because of digital imaging systems the parameters that are used to acquire an image can vary. Therefore protocols for testing each piece of equipment will need to be drawn up locally utilising factors that are in everyday use.

The following outlines a larger range of tests that can be carried out.

Grey scale level reproduction
e.g. Leeds test object GS2

This test tool has a step wedge within it of ten equal steps in contrast. Also included are disks of material with a contrast difference of 0 & 10% and 90% & 99%. The step wedge should appear on the resultant image as covering the full grey scale of the system. If this is not the case, then either the imaging system is not able to perceive this grey scale (unlikely) or the preset parameters for displaying the images are not appropriate and should be altered.

Low Contrast Test
e.g. Leeds test object N3

This test tool contains 11 mm diameter discs of a range of different X-ray contrast values. Contrast values decrease towards the centre of the test object. Noise within the system will result in the degradation of low contrast difference and the amount of noise will determine at what point the circles are no longer visible. Viewers can convert number of details seen to threshold contrast values using a data table.

Minimum visible detail contrast test
e.g. Leeds test object TO10

This is similar to N3 in that it contains circular details of various X-ray contrast values. However, in this test object the details also vary in size from 11 mm diameter to 0.25 mm diameter. This allows the system to be assessed for its threshold contrast for different object sizes.

Limiting Resolution
e.g. Huttner type 18 test object

This test tool is comprised of a square wave patterns (line pair per millimetre – lp/mm ranging from 0.5 lp/mm to 5 lp/mm. By using a table to refer to the last lp/mm visible by an experienced observer the limiting resolution of the system can be evaluated.

Exposure Ranges
All of the imaging systems currently on the market offer some way of indicating whether the imaging plate has received an exposure which is within an acceptable range for the system and the examination that is being carried out. That is not to say that the system is unable to operate outside this range. A computed radiography cassette could be many times over exposed and still manage to produce an acceptable image.

The danger exists that all exposures are set high to ensure that all images are produced with a good SNR. If this occurs the change to digital imaging will result in an increase in dose.

A random check on a sample of images everyday to ensure that they are within the exposure range suggested by the manufacturer is advised. Regular dosimetry should still be carried out in conjunction with the local Medical Physics department. It is also important to ensure that all staff are aware that they should be using the exposures provided on the exposure charts (allowing for a small degree of interpretation for patient size).

Automatic Exposure Chambers
In addition, when the CR system is installed it is likely that the operation of AEC systems will require adjustment (by x-ray equipment service engineers) to ensure performance is optimised for use with CR.

CONCLUSION

Image quality assurance in computed radiography and digital imaging is difficult due to the variable response of the imaging system but current test tools can be used to provide meaningful evaluation of equipment. This is providing that appropriate tests have first been carried out on the visual display unit being used for assessment.

SAMPLE REGIME FOR QA

This is not intended to be a gold standard, but is a suggested framework that a department might build upon to establish their own comprehensive regime of tests.

The above list is from the BIR publication "Assurance of Quality in the Diagnostic Imaging Department" 2nd Edition (published in 2001).

It is very likely to that a list of tests similar to this will appear in the next revision of IPEM 77 when digital radiography is included.

Table 2 – Example of Routine Quality Assurance

Test	Frequency
Exposure Index Monitoring	3 monthly
Clinical exposure index monitoring	3 monthly
Low contrast resolution	6 monthly
Spatial resolution limit	6 monthly
AEC sensitivity	3 monthly

REFERENCES AND SOURCES

BOOKS

Carter P.H. (Ed.) 1994 Chesneys' Equipment for Student Radiographers Blackwell Scientific Publications

Chesney D.N., Chesney M.O. 1984 **X-ray Equipment for Student Radiographers** Blackwell Scientific Publications

Forster E. 1986 **Equipment for Diagnostic Radiography** MTP Press Ltd

Gunn C. 1995 **Radiographic Imaging** Churchill Livingstone

Hiles P.A., Starrit H.C. 1996 **Measurement of the Performance Characteristics of Diagnostic X-ray Systems Used In Medicine – Part II – X-ray II and television**, Institution of Engineering in Medicine and Biology, York

Hill D.R. 1984 **Principles of Diagnostic X-ray Apparatus** Philips Technical Library

Huang H.K.1996 **PACS in Biomedical Imaging** VCH

ICRU 1995 **Medical Imaging – The Assessment of Image Quality** International Commission on radiation Units and Measurements

K-Care 1992 **MDD/92/36** Medical devices Directorate

Li Evans A. 1981 **The Evaluation of Medical Images Medical Physics Handbooks (10)** Adam Hilger Ltd

Stockley S.M. 1986 **A manual of Radiographic Equipment** Churchill Livingstone

Wilks R. 1987 **Principles of Radiological Physics** Churchill Livingstone

WWW

http://www.dsclabs.com/smpte_article.htm
  Information on all types of test tools for monitor evaluation.

http://www.smpte.org/
  Official site of the Society of Motion Picture and Television Engineers

http://www.ipem.org.uk
  Institute of Physics and Engineering in Medicine

http://www.nottingham.ac.uk/physics/ugrad/courses/mod_home/f33ab5/notes/Image.doc
  Information on image parameters

http://www.lxi.leeds.ac.uk/TestObjects/index.htm
  Test objects homepage. Large amounts of useful information, tutorials and references

http://www.dundee.ac.uk/medphys/documents/balqual.pdf
  PDF on image quality from the physicists perspective

http://www.kcare.co.uk/
  MDA site for X-ray equipment

http://www.pacsnet.org.uk/
  MDA site specific to PACS

10: COMMON PRESET FUNCTIONS AND PARAMETERS

Jason Oakley

INTRODUCTION

Chapter eight, Image Processing laid out the basics on image formation and manipulation in mathematical terms. Chapter Nine – Image quality sought to define what image quality constituted and how it could be measured. This chapter will look at how image manipulation and adjustment of the factors that make up image quality can be used as an aid to interpretation and diagnosis of radiological images.

Once again this book will not cover what might be considered traditional digital imaging techniques such as digital subtraction angiography (DSA), but will focus on the newer plain radiography imaging systems, although many of these factors will apply equally to other modalities.

The reason that preset functions and parameters have been chosen is that they can be easily explained and demonstrated on images. User controlled variables are equally diverse and several of these will be included for completeness if they are part of the automatic set up of the system.

This chapter will be based on the FUJI Computed Radiography system and the parameters that are available for image adjustment on the Fuji QA (Quality Assurance) -WS771 QA Workstation and the Fuji HI-C655 Reporting Workstation. It will first cover image manipulations that can be carried out prior to reporting on the QA Workstation.

FUJI QA-WS771QA WORKSTATION

The QA workstation is designed to be used by the radiographer or radiologist for the approval of an image before sending to the reporting workstation. However it should be borne in mind that the system should be set up to automatically process every image to be of optimal quality. If you find that nearly all images produced require some form of manipulation then it is very likely that the preset manipulations carried out after acquisition are inaccurate and adjustment should be made.

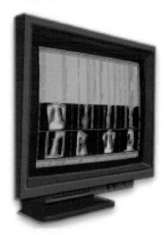

Figure 1 – Fuji QA-WS771 QA Workstation
(picture courtesy of Fuji)

There are several key functions instantly available for adjusting image quality.

BRIGHTNESS CONTRAST CONTROL

These functions are controlled by moving the mouse over the image, left click and holding, which changes the mouse icon from a small arrow to a horizontal and vertical set of arrows. Holding the left hand mouse button down and moving left to right adjusts the brightness of the image. Holding the left hand mouse button down and moving up and down alters the contrast of the image.

If the monitor is correctly adjusted then these functions should be all that is required to adjust an image slightly to improve the subjective viewing of the image. It is for this reason that everyday adjustment of the monitor contrast and brightness must not be made.

DEMOGRAPHIC ALTERATION

As with conventional film every step should be taken to ensure that any radiographic image acquired has all of the correct information on it from the start. However if an error is made and the person that took the image is 100% sure that the image is that of their patient then the facility exists to alter the patient information contained within the image. This includes access to the name, date of birth, hospital number and other data stored in free text fields.

Any such changes to patient information must be trackable; that is the alterations made to the patient information should be easily attributable to the person who made the changes.

IMAGE ANNOTATION

Image annotation has always been an important part of radiography. With conventional film it was very easy to take a permanent marker and record pertinent information such as patient position and exposure on a film. With a digital image this is equally important.

The FUJI system does not allow free text writing on the screen but comes with numerous preset terms such as kV, mAs, AP Erect etc, as well as a complete set of numbers and letters that will cover the multitude of annotation requirements. These are in the form of bitmaps that can be embedded in the image (be permanently placed into whilst not being part of that image).

This method can also be used to ensure that correct anatomical markers are visible on an image, although every effort should still be made to ensure that a radiographer identifiable marker is visible on every image.

The annotations stored with the image are in the form of bitmaps, that is a file that tends to already be fairly pixelated. If your images are going to be compressed at all it is worth testing the compression on images that have been annotated to ensure that any subsequent compression does not render the text unreadable.

AUTOMATIC SHUTTERING

Whilst accurate collimation is of the utmost importance in good radiographic technique, this is particularly true for CR. The white borders that are left around the image do in fact distract the eye from the detail within the image itself. This phenomena has been tackled in conventional radiography with the use of cut outs of black card, automatically collimating viewing boxes and other ingenious methods.

With digital imaging this can be done by the computer, blacking out any areas that might

have appeared white. This function has been utilised for many years in the laser printing of computed tomography (CT) images.

The area to be blacked out can either be designated by the user or set as an automatic function. In the case of a manual change the facility to preview the end result is given prior to the change being made permanent. Figures 2a and 2b show the difference between a shuttered and an unshuttered image.

There is a difference in the maximum density achieved via exposure and the maximum density achieved by computer blacking out and this allows the viewer to discern where the original

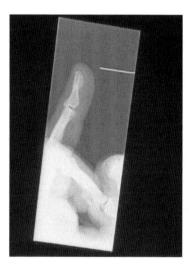

Figure 2a – Unshuttered image

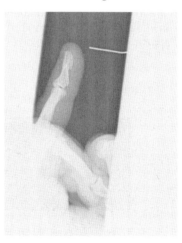

Figure 2b – Shuttered image

collimation marks were. Shuttering should not be used to hide poor collimation as a result of poor radiographic technique.

IMAGE ORIENTATION

When reading an image plate any system will read it in a regular fashion, starting on one edge, and finishing on the opposite edge. The image will then be displayed in this orientation unless told other wise. The FUJI system allows image orientation to be attached to the cassette along with patient information, but this is often programmed incorrectly or technique dictates an unusual orientation of the cassette.

To counter this, retrospective rotation of the image can be carried out at the QA workstation to ensure that all images are viewed in the correct way.

FUJI HI-C655 REPORTING WORKSTATION FUNCTIONS

Other than a complex search interface that allows the user to find the images they wish to look at by looking for a wide number of different parameters (such as patient name, date of birth, hospital number etc) the rest of the available functions are to do with image manipulation.

When an image is displayed a 'toolbox' can be made to appear (figure 4). This toolbox contains

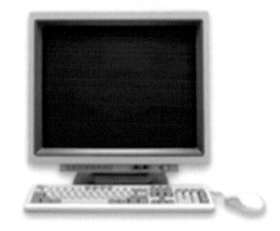

Figure 3 – Fuji HI-C655 Reporting Workstation

'buttons' that when pressed carry out a certain function automatically. Each of these functions will be looked at in turn.

PRESET MANIPULATIONS

The first five buttons in the top row are preset image manipulations that have been chosen by the users as the most useful for their needs. These are not rigid, and can be changed to suit any particular need or department. The effects will be compared against figure 5, which shows the original image.

This Image has already undergone some automatic processing in order to display it to what is considered the optimal quality. The appearance can be dictated by the users

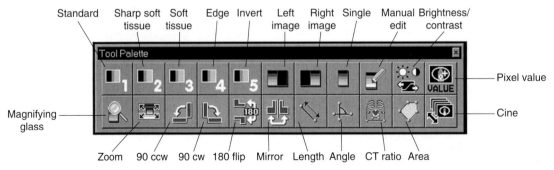

Figure 4 – Toolbox with functions labelled

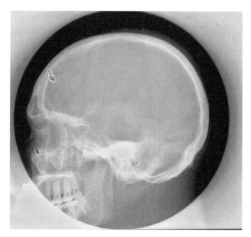

Figure 5 – Original image

through pre-programming of the algorithms that are attached to the image when it is named.

The look up table (LUT) for the response of the storage plate to exposure is shown in figure 6. This is typical sigmoid curve.

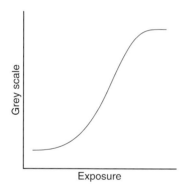

Figure 6 – Response cure for original image

This curve produces the histogram shown in figure 7.

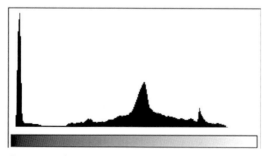

Figure 7 – Histogram for normal image

This histogram demonstrates the lack of actual 'white' in the image and the peaks around nearly black and mid-grey.

Preset Manipulation One

Preset manipulation one is a 'standard' image filter that very slightly softens the image by reducing the peaks slightly to make the image comparable to all other images. This is again programmed in by the users on installation (see figure 8).

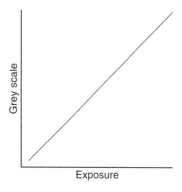

Figure 8 – Preset manipulation one

The response curve for this image (figure 9) is a straight line which mimics the typical response of a storage phosphor plate to exposure.

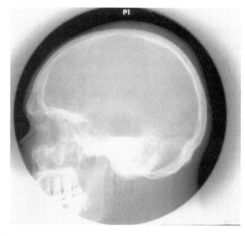

Figure 9 – Response curve for preset manipulation one

The histogram (figure 10) shows that the peaks have been reduced to produce a softer image.

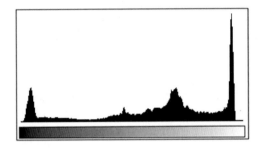

Figure 10 – Histogram for preset manipulation one

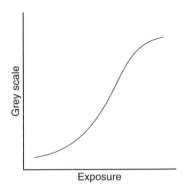

Figure 12 – Response curve for manipulation two

Preset Manipulation Two

This manipulation is designed to accentuate the soft tissue present with the image, so is essentially a softening filter, which reduces the contrast in the image (figure 11).

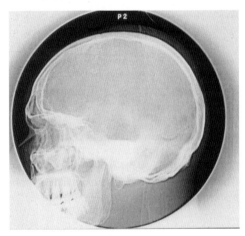

Figure 11 – Preset manipulation two

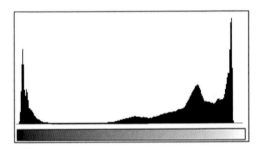

Figure 13 – Histogram for preset manipulation two

Preset Manipulation Three

Preset manipulation three is a soft tissue enhancement without the edge detection so the bony structure appear very indistinct (figure 14).

The trabecular bone is far less detailed and the skin border clearer. The response curve (figure 12) shows a sigmoid curve that is slightly flatter than the original, reducing the contrast to reveal soft tissue detail.

The histogram (figure 13) shows that the peaks seen in the first two images have been broadened to reduce the contrast in the image. The histogram also reveals that a certain amount of edge enhancement has been applied in order to more clearly define any foreign bodies that might be within the tissues.

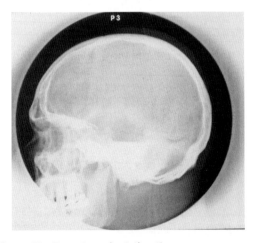

Figure 14 – Preset manipulation three

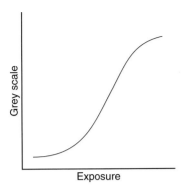

Figure 15 – Response curve for preset manipulation three

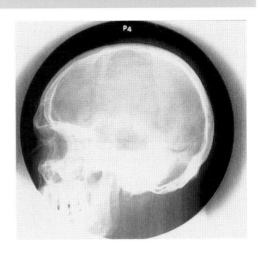

Figure 17 – Preset manipulation four

The histogram (figure 16) clearly shows the difference between preset manipulation two, where the difference in the smaller peaks had been accentuated. Here the histogram shows a much smoother and flatter profile.

The response curve (figure 18) shows how the contrast has been improved in the central region of the curve, but lessened at either end. This results in a high contrast image with accentuated detail

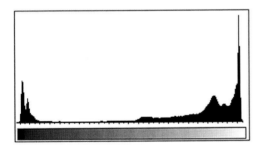

Figure 16 – Histogram for preset manipulation three

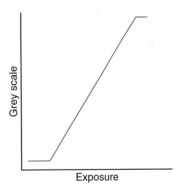

Figure 18 – Response curve for preset manipulation four

Preset Manipulation Four

Preset manipulation four is an algorithm designed to enhance the fine bony detail in the image (figure 17). The trabeculae are very clear and a certain amount of sharpening has been applied. This can make the image less pleasing to the eye but does in fact aid diagnosis.

The histogram (figure 19) demonstrates the separating out of the data around clear peaks.

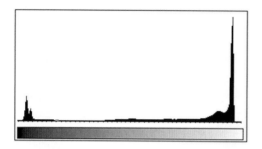

Figure 19 – Histogram for preset manipulation four

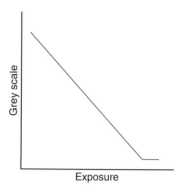

Figure 21 – Response curve for preset manipulation five

Preset Manipulation Five

Preset manipulation five is an inverting algorithm that reverses the grey scale on the image. Whilst this does not inherently change the detail of emphasise for structures within the image it does alter the way the mind looks at the image and can be enough to confirm an interpretation or diagnosis. Other functions can be built into this function and in this case edge enhancement is also included. Figure 20 shows the manipulated image.

The histogram (figure 22) shows the reversal of light and dark, with most of the pixel values clustered towards the white end of the grey scale.

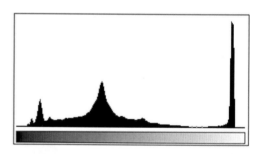

Figure 22 – Histogram for preset manipulation five

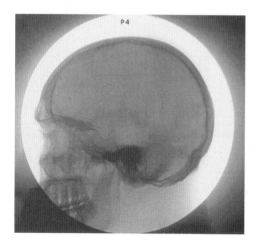

Figure 20 – Preset manipulation five

The response curve for this is again a straight line but it is in the opposite direction to preset manipulation one (figure 21).

LEFT IMAGE AND RIGHT IMAGE

This function is used when it might be useful to compare the same image side-by-side under two different manipulations. These buttons can be preset by the user on installation with any manipulation (such as edge enhancement and inversion) to allow quick manipulation and viewing of images.

SINGLE

The single button undoes all of the manipulation that has been performed on the image at the workstation and returns it to its original state.

MANUAL EDIT

This allows more experienced users to enter a sub screen for direct input of parameters to alter the images appearances. This tends not to be intuitive as manipulating the image in real time but can be useful in developing new algorithms to manipulated images for specific functions.

BRIGHTNESS AND CONTRAST

This button triggers the mouse to act horizontally as a brightness control and vertically as a contrast control. A combination of these can help to make an image look subjectively better.

PIXEL VALUE

This function allows the user to hover over a given area and the value of the pixel as a grey scale number will be given.

MAGNIFYING GLASS

This function introduces a box onto the main image that contains a magnified view of the area underneath of it. The size of this box may be altered, as indeed may the level of magnification. Once the user is happy with these two settings the resulting box may then be moved around the image like a magnifying glass.

ZOOM

Zoom allows the user to select the magnitude to which the whole image will be magnified. This will result in only a portion of the image being visible on the screen at any one time. The image can be 'grabbed' using the mouse and scrolled around the screen to reveal the entire image.

90CCW, 90CW AND 180 FLIP

The difficulties of orientating an imaging plate have been mentioned previously. The first two buttons allow the image to be rotated 90 degrees either to the left or the right. The 180 flip button allows the image to be rotated 180 degrees at the click of the mouse. These functions allow the image to be viewed in the plane that is best suited to the viewer.

MIRROR

The mirror function allows the image to be 'turned around', that is left becomes right and vice versa. This might be used if an image had been read as antero-posterior (AP) but had in fact been taken postero-anterior (PA). This sort of manipulation should of course be used with care to avoid missing conditions such as os situs invertus or cardio-dextra.

LENGTH

The length function allows the distance between two points to be measured. The resulting measurement is displayed in centimetres. However allowances for magnification within the image must be taken into account.

ANGLE

The angle function can be used to measure the angle between any two lines that bisect each other. This is useful in assessing features such as Bohler's angle in the Calcaneum.

CARDIO THORACIC RATIO (CTR)

This function allows the user to measure the widest point of the chest and then the widest point for the heart. These distances and the ratio between them is then displayed on the screen.

These two factors allow the cardio-thoracic ratio to be established which is a good indicator of the level of cardio-megaly present in the patient.

AREA

The area function allows a perimeter to be drawn around an object and the area of this object to be calculated.

CINE

The cine function is used when the workstation is being used to view multiple images that have a spatial or temporal record associated with them. This would include computed tomography (CT) images, magnetic resonance images (MRI) and digital angiography images. The cine feature allows these images to be rapidly displayed to give the feeling of movement. This function is only active if the DICOM component for this function is installed on the worksation.

CONCLUSIONS

All systems will have different features that will allow the user to manipulate the image that is in front of them easier and faster. In general these manipulations or functions can be determined by the users and can reduce the amount of time spent manipulating individual images. If the original algorithms for the display of the initial image have been carefully selected the number of images requiring manipulation, and thus extra time spent on them will be minimal, and these changes will be made for diagnostic purposes rather than for quality reasons.

11: PRACTICAL EXPERIENCES OF USING COMPUTED AND DIGITAL RADIOGRAPHY EQUIPMENT

Jason Oakley and Martin Benwell

INTRODUCTION

Many of the preceding chapters have dealt with technical issues surrounding computer systems within hospital environments. This chapter is designed to expound on the practical experiences of those who have actually used computer systems within hospital environments. The information included had been drawn from the collective experience of the authors and their colleagues.

This may help to prevent other departments from 'reinventing the wheel', or at least from inventing it square.

TRAINING ISSUES

Most radiographers are now used to change in both their working practice and their working environment. However it should not be assumed that all staff will cope with the change from existing practices to the use of technology.

It is not that long ago that day sheets were still used to record the patients that were attending for procedures that day. This was a simple tool that only required the ability to write legibly and, if stored in a logical fashion, fulfilled its main purpose of recording data that could be used at a later date if necessary.

The change to a radiology information system (RIS) has enabled this information to be more accessible, and if properly designed the system should be able to deliver almost any combination of facts about the demographics of patients attending etc.

The installation of a RIS has far reaching effects within a radiology department, affecting all members of staff from the ground up. This means that there are a wide range of individuals, with varying levels of education and experience to be considered. A standard training programme is essential, but this should not be a one-stop shop. It should be the first part of an ongoing programme of refreshers and updates that can allow staff to improve gradually.

As with many computer applications software some part of the RIS will be very easy to pick up, and these key functions will be used by most people. The more advance functions take longer to become familiar with and it is these points that ongoing training can strengthen.

A method of monitoring the system is also essential to identify what is going wrong and why. This can aid the trainers in tailoring the training to meet the demands of their staff. What must also be in place is an atmosphere of genuine support within the department. This is the only way that staff who are struggling with the system can be expected to be effectively identified and helped.

The same applies to the introduction of new imaging systems, either computed or digital. Whilst the main impact will be on the radiographic staff, it will not stop there. For example one of the traditional roles of the radiographic helper has been in the sorting of minor problems with processing equipment in order that the radiographers can continue to carry out radiographic procedures whilst they attempt to restore the processor to working order.

In some departments this role has been naturally extended to the sorting of minor problems with the imaging equipment. As with most computer systems a problem is often simple and can be solved with a reboot of that or another piece of equipment. This does not negate the need for an overall administrator (to be discussed) but means that they can be kept free to carry out other duties.

It has been assumed that all radiographers are computer literate to some degree but this is not the case. The Government recognises the need for a certain level of literacy in the NHS and it is intended that all staff, regardless of grade, should complete the European Computer Driving Licence (ECDL) that will give them basic computer skills.

Until this level of competency has been achieved all staff should be approached as novices. An air of openness can also help those who require further help to come forward, and these staff must be supported in their training.

ACCEPTANCE ISSUES

Change is never readily accepted, as scepticism tends to dominate and leads to all those involved focussing on the negative side of any situation. With hindsight groups may reflect that the change was for the best, and that they are glad that the change took place, but at the time any change in working practices may be seen as another inconvenience in a working environment that is already at breaking point.

This will obviously trouble those who are not sure of the benefits to themselves and their colleagues through their involvement in the project. This book is not designed to impart management training but there are several key points that experience has shown are of great importance.

- Appoint an overall systems administrator at an early stage.
- Early consultation. The earlier that staff who are to be affected by the implementation of new technology are involved the more likely they are to accept the change. This can be for many reasons, including ownership of the change, but also because they are likely to be more willing to try the change out in view of their consultation. This applies equally to different groups of staff.
- Rather than telling people what they are going to get, find out what they want and establish whether it is achievable. It is also important to know why they think a certain factor is important. If it would be 'nice' if a piece of equipment did something, then it is not essential. If the person's job cannot be completed without a function then it becomes essential
- Teamwork. Build a team of 'super users' who can help with the day-to-day problems and advice that the staff will generate. This shares responsibility.
- Listen to the many, and not the few. It is often the case that one or two people will make the most noise about the implementation of a new system. It is important that when issues arise it is established whether this is the opinion of the larger group, or just the few who are willing to be vocal about their feelings. That is not to say that they should be ignored because there must be issues to be resolved.

COMPLIANCE ISSUES

Whereas acceptance of a system can be difficult it is also possible for those using a system to accept it but then fail to comply with acceptable methods of working practice. This is not a new problem and should not entirely be associated with the use of new technologies.

In example let us consider a conventional x-ray film. It is accepted practice to ensure that the correct name, patient details, marker etc are on the film and are clearly visible. If any of these are missing then each department will have an accepted practice that allows the film to be corrected, or if there is any doubt, for the patient to be re x-rayed. Whilst these practices exist and are accepted by the staff, it does not necessarily follow that they are implemented on a rigorous basis. Films will get put through with the wrong marker or wrong name, and it is through the use of effective safety nets (such as quality assurance and reporting) that mistakes are avoided.

Checking the important details on a conventional film should be relatively easy, but in a digital environment this may be very different. On many workstations the name of the patient is not instantly obvious and may require a separate screen of patient details to be accessed. This may mean that the image is assessed for its quality and position, but the patient details are not checked as rigorously as they should be.

ORIENTATION

Orientation of images is really another compliance issue. When an image is acquired the computer has to be told the orientation of the cassette. Most departments will have a standard protocol for positioning patients, such as the green end of the cassette to the patients right or cephalic. This can then be used to tell the computer which way to display the image.

However, one of the skills of radiography is being able to adapt to different situations and this means that it is common for the orientation of the cassette to be altered. The computer can easily be informed of the change of direction, but this takes time and thought to do so.

Once the image has been read by the computer, and subsequently displayed the radiographer has another chance to re-orientate the image, but again this takes time and may again not be done. The images subsequently get sent to the network orientated inappropriately. The knock on effect is that every person who subsequently views the image will have to re-orientate it to look at it in the standard anatomical position.

It would be more time effective if the image was stored in the correct orientation initially. This also reflects better on the department as a whole.

THE RADIOGRAPHER AS A COMPUTER EXPERT

The PACS within a hospital is generally a global solution to imaging, and may be run by the imaging department, computer services, medical physics or a dedicated unit of people. However, the primary role of the PACS will be seen as the display of x-ray images and this will mean that the perceived owners of the system will be the x-ray department.

So when the system goes down, or images cannot be found the first step is often to contact the x-ray department for help. This is compounded in scenarios such as Accident and Emergency where radiographers are generally on hand 24 hours per day. This has led some departments to ensure that the radiographers in these areas are able to deal with minor problems by carrying out protocol led checks.

This might include being trained to carryout the standard computer solution of shutting down and re-booting the system, checking for memory shortages etc. Whilst this may be yet another role for the radiographer to perform it can help the department in the long run by increasing other user acceptance of the wider radiology imaging provision.

It is important to remember that this provision should not replace the full support of the PACS, but is rather a safety net for simple problems that might otherwise take a long time to sort out and cost a potentially large call out fee. A typical example that the author has been called to many times is the storage of the keyboard on a primarily mouse driven image viewing program. Because the keyboard is not needed (except on start up for password entering) the tendency was to place it on top of the monitor. Throughout the day it would get knocked behind the monitor and the keys would become depressed. This would lock the system up and moments later the doctors would report that the system had 'gone down'. This problem was easily remedied but did increase the perception of the radiographers as computer experts.

CONTINGENCY PLANS

This is a very important area for imaging departments. If there is one department that the hospital cannot be without for any period of time it is the imaging department. There is little that the imaging department would have been able to do in a total power cut anyway, and it is up to the Estates department to ensure that adequate backup is provided during a power grid failure.

What the imaging department must ensure is that all of the essential equipment is protected from power interruption by a UPS (uninterruptible power supply) and that the power to this equipment is on the backup supply.

However the digital imaging department also has several other areas that have to be considered. Firstly what will happen if the hospital network goes down for any reason? It is essential that, if the network fails, the imaging department can still function as a stand-alone network. This can be achieved by either having the department as a true sub-network or by utilising a backup hub that allows the equipment to be connected as a local network in an emergency situation.

The other issue in this scenario is how is the rest of the hospital going to view the images during this down time? Whilst the hospital may have been striving to be totally filmless, provision must be made to have the ability to print hard copies of some description.

SECURITY ISSUES

These are many-fold, and can have an effect on the working practices of departments. For example every time a user interacts with a terminal they should log on and once finished they should log off. This has time implications in a busy department and is a source of frustration to the staff. Systems can be set up to log off automatically after a user, but this again can cause frustration. One solution is a generic log on for an area but this will reduce your ability to track which individuals have carried out an examination and leave the system open to abuse.

Levels of access need to be decided upon in order to ensure that the information an individual is able to access can be justified under the terms of the Data Protection Act 1998. Data that is termed as 'sensitive' should be particularly protected.

Can people who are not meant to see them see any of the monitors? If so, this has implications under the Data Protection Act of 1998 as well, as non-authorised individuals might be able to view data that they should not.

These are just a few of the security issues that departments must consider.

PRACTICAL EXPERIENCES OF REPORTING FROM SOFT COPY IMAGES

This section has been written from a pilot study conducted using both reporting radiographers and consultant radiologists. It is designed to give the reader an honest opinion from the experiences of those who are currently extensively using softcopy technologies to report images.

The results will be listed under the questions that were asked and the responses of the two groups compared if differences were noted. The questionnaire was designed with the help of several of the other authors and then tested on a small trial group prior to being issued with departmental permission to those involved in softcopy reporting.

The term softcopy refers to radiographs obtained on a computed radiography (CR) system and the term hardcopy refers to radiographs obtained using a conventional film/screen combination.

Thanks are due to the staff at both Queen Alexandra and St Mary's hospitals in Portsmouth, Hampshire.

How long have you been reporting from softcopy?

The mean length of experience of softcopy reporting for all respondents was 2.5 years. The consultants had on average 2.7 years experience and the radiographers had 2 years experience. Although the radiologists had slightly more experience the difference was not statistically significant.

Is softcopy reporting easier than hardcopy reporting and if so why?

The answer from the radiologists was a unanimous yes. 100% of the respondents found the system easier to use and the main reasons given were:

- Faster reporting – no need to take films out of packets to find the latest image
- Automatic work lists that allow just the relevant patients to be pulled and viewed in rapid succession
- Less loss of information (films, reports etc.)
- Ability to manipulate the image, such as brightness and contrast adjustment

The radiographers agreed on the whole with the above list but added that for single images hardcopy and softcopy were very similar. It was also noted that at times confidence in a report could be increased by viewing the final hardcopy. This was demonstrated by the fact that many more hard copies were requested in the initial days of the CR system when confidence in the softcopy technology was at its lowest.

Is softcopy reporting more efficient than hardcopy reporting and if so why?

Again the radiologists gave a 100% yes to this question and two main reasons were given for the increase in efficiency:

- Removal of the time taken to get films out of the packets and find the appropriate film
- Rapid display of the next image for reporting

The radiographers gave slightly different reasons;

- No time wasted looking through packets for images, and images should never be 'lost'
- Image manipulation means that whilst you could theoretically spend longer looking at an image, you actually come to your decision far quicker and with more confidence. This confidence seems to come from the perception that manipulating an image is equivalent to looking at a number of images.

A valid comment was that an increase in efficiency at this part of the reporting chain might have a limited effect on the overall efficiency. Whilst the radiologists and radiographers were able to report more images, this led to an increased amount of work for the clerical staff. This then necessitates the need for voice recognition systems to remove another link from the reporting chain and improve efficiency even more.

In your experience which is of higher quality, soft or hardcopy, and why?

This question produced differing opinions in both groups. The radiologists who felt that hardcopy was best (28%) gave exactly the same reason. This was that CR technology compensated for poor radiography, but if too low an exposure was given then the image looked superficially acceptable, but the detail in the image suffered.

Those that felt softcopy was better quoted that the ability to manipulate the images, revealing more of the information within the image, increased the images quality. It was recorded by one radiologist that certain modalities had always been reported from the screen, such as ultrasound (US) and that this was now becoming the norm for computed tomography (CT) and (MRI), and that it was a confidence issue as well as a quality issue.

Interestingly, the radiographers felt that one of the reasons why softcopy was better was the fact that an over or under exposure was compensated for by the system. This is in contrast to the radiologists' viewpoint that this is actually a problem.

It was also noted that whilst hardcopy could be theoretically of a higher quality it would be difficult to obtain an image that demonstrated both bony and soft tissue detail in the way that a digital film could.

Which, given the preference, would you rather report from (hard or softcopy) and why?

Despite the last question demonstrating that some of the individuals did have an issue with the quality of the images 100% of the respondents stated that they would rather report from softcopy if given the option. The reasons given were:

- Ability to manipulate the image
- Ability to zoom the image
- Increased speed of reporting

- Less handling of film packets
- Better quality

The only caveat was that chest x-rays should still be reported from film as the respondent felt that there was no monitor that could do a full size chest x-ray justice.

How has softcopy reporting affected your workload?

This question produced a wide range of responses from the groups involved. The radiologists firstly noted that they were able to report faster and thus the total turn around time was quicker. However, previously to CR many films produced went with the patient and subsequently were returned too late for a report to be of any importance and were thus not reported.

With the introduction of CR the images are all available so they should all be reported. This means that the actual workload of the department has increased significantly.

A major issue at the present time when many of the patient's previous images are on hardcopy is the time spent trying to compare a softcopy image with a previous hardcopy image. As time goes by this will occur less and less but should be a consideration for any hospital introducing digital imaging systems.

The radiographers on the whole agreed with these comments, noting that it made 'hot' reporting in the accident and emergency (A&E) situation a reality.

In your experience what are the main benefits of softcopy reporting?

This question produced some overlap with other questions, but some new points also emerged:

- Ability to manipulate images
- No lost images
- Ability to display multiple images for comparison
- Increased speed in reporting
- Leaner working environment with no packets

In your experience what are the main benefits of hardcopy reporting?

Hardcopy still has a place and the respondents

clearly felt that there were several advantages to hardcopy that will persist:

- Old films available in the same format
- No pixelation of images
- Increased image quality (theoretical)
- Easier to compare with old images
- Manual measurements very easy
- Easier to compare lots of images on a bank of viewing boxes
- Better resolution for chest x-rays
- Portable and utilises low cost equipment to view
- Something about having a physical image to look at

In your experience what are the main disadvantages of softcopy reporting?

The next two questions were asked because it does not necessarily follow that the advantages of one system are the disadvantages of another. Again a wide number of responses were returned:

- Old images not available in the same format
- Not always clear when an old image isn't present
- Not always obvious that more than one image is present for the same examination
- Pixelation at high magnification
- Capability of system to attempt to rectify poor radiography leading to grainy images
- If an image is named incorrectly it can be nearly impossible to find
- Artefacts can degrade the image
- More difficult to compare to old films
- Often not enough workstations to allow multiple images to be compared
- Often not enough high quality workstations to allow reporting at busy times

In your experience what are the main disadvantages of hardcopy reporting?

Interestingly the disadvantages of hardcopy are nearly all its shortcoming when compared to softcopy, and not problems specific to hardcopy technologies:

- Unable to manipulate the images
- Soft tissues and bone not visible in equal amounts

- Takes longer to find the image you require
- Handling packets and paper reports is very time consuming
- Film storage is a big problem
- Lost images and delay in getting old films

What problems have you encountered whilst soft copy reporting?

Both groups found the main problem to be the accurate pulling of work lists prior to reporting. This is an administration issue and whilst a minor one the break in work flow was considered distracting and could result in the report being issued on the wrong patient.

Other areas highlighted were:

- Lack of access to a workstation to report
- Lost images
- The computers seem slow to respond once you have got used to them meaning that the efficiency of the system is being reduced by the technology
- Some J-Peg artefacts visible on older images post long term storage
- Poor quality radiography, but not sure if this is specific to CR

How do you see the future of radiology in the digital era?

This question produced a very positive response towards the technology:

- Essential that radiography moves forward with the available technology
- It is the way forward and the sooner the better
- Improved reporting conditions
- PACS everywhere – truly filmless
- Digital screening
- Nationwide specialist referral via telemedicine links
- Global review of medical indemnity to allow international consultation

Which technologies do you see as having the biggest impact on your role?

The radiographers all considered this to be PACS, teleradiology and new digital acquisition media.

The radiologists listed several different areas:

- Increased speed of networks, processors and increased archives
- More radiographer role expansion
- Digital radiography
- Voice recognition reporting systems
- PACS

Any other comments you would like to make?

No significantly different comments were made by any of the respondents.

CONCLUSION

Despite the unavoidable problems that come with the initiation of any new system the common consensus is that once you have experienced computed radiography systems and become accustomed to their nuances there is no turning back. The advantages outweigh the disadvantages and it should be remembered that this is an emerging technology that means that theoretically things will get better.

In the words of one of the respondents, despite all of the problems, the digital future is bright.

12: SUMMARY OF IMPORTANT DOCUMENTS

Jason Oakley

INTRODUCTION

The aim of this book was not to turn its readers into computer engineers, nor to make them completely proficient in all aspects of digital medical imaging. Its primary aim was to provide enough knowledge to give the reader an effective grounding in digital medical imaging. What it cannot hope to achieve is to impart the entire vast amount of accessory information that is available and may well be needed in the development of any digital radiology provision.

This is primarily because there is a plethora of documents that relate both directly and indirectly to digital medical imaging and information technology within the National Health Service (NHS) . To address this mountain of potential information this chapter will briefly outline the contents of some of the documents that it is useful for the modern practitioner to be aware of. This chapter is not designed to replace the documents and it would be wise for the readers to obtain and read them if pertinent. The comments are the author's interpretation of the documents.

The aim of this section is designed to enable you to know where the information that you require can be found.

Where the documents are available on the Internet appropriate URLs have been included, but as always these will only remain active for a certain time. Many sites also state that the definitive document is the official printed and bound version.

Certain websites and the resources that they contain will also be discussed where appropriate.

This section will further be divided into two sections. The first will deal with documents that refer to areas both inside and outside of the NHS (General Documents) and the second section documents that are specific to the NHS.

There are three main types of documents that you will come across.

1. Regulations (sometimes called acts) are the actual laws, and these will be extensive and more often than not, far from being easy reading.
2. Guidance notes are the interpretation of the regulations into an easier to understand format, but do not replace the regulations as the legal document.
3. Codes of practice are the practical examples of good working methods in a specific working area.

GENERIC DOCUMENTS

DATA PROTECTION ACT 1998

Source: www.dataprotection.gov.uk

This revision of the previous Data Protection Act (1984) has enlarged its scope to cover the protection of all data that is stored on individuals and no longer refers only to data stored on computers. It is based on European directives that set out to ensure the security of information whilst also ensuring that the information can be sent freely for legitimate purposes.

All individuals must be made aware of all of the purposes that their information might be used for and agree to it being used for those purposes. Individuals must now give informed consent, rather than having to say that they wish not to have their data used for such purposes.

Every establishment, including hospitals, should have a Data Protection Officer who is knowledgeable about the Data Protection Act. Any uses of patient information should be registered with them to ensure that the Data Protection Act is not being contravened in any way. They in turn will refer to the Governments Data Protection Registrar should the need arise.

To fully understand the data protection act it is worth obtaining the full explanation of the principles and the full document. These, used in conjunction with each other, can answer most queries that arise, but another source of information should be the data protection officer to whom the modern imaging department should become a familiar area.

The Data Protection Act can be explained via eight general principles, which have been quoted from www.dataprotection.gov.uk. From here the full document and other associated documents can be downloaded.

Principle 1 – "**Personal data shall be processed fairly and lawfully and, in particular, shall not be processed unless –**

- **at least one of the conditions in Schedule 2 is met, and**
- **in the case of sensitive personal data, at least one of the conditions in Schedule 3 is also met."**

Schedule two lists the extensive reasons for which information can be legally stored. Schedule three identifies what is considered to be sensitive data, such as race or political beliefs, and the reasons for which this may be stored, but only with the individuals explicit consent.

Principle 2 – **"Personal data shall be obtained only for one or more specified and lawful purposes, and shall not be further processed in any manner incompatible with that purpose or those purposes."**

This principle states that it is no longer enough merely to register the information that you want to record and get an individuals permission to record it. There must be valid reasons to record it.

Principle 3 – **"Personal data shall be adequate, relevant and not excessive in relation to the purpose or purposes for which they are processed."**

It is important that you record enough information for the purpose for which you need it. For example a name is no good without at least a date of birth. In the same way there would be no requirement within an x-ray department to know the name of a persons dog, so this information would be excessive and also not relevant.

Principle 4 – **"Personal data shall be accurate and, where necessary, kept up to date".**

There is no point in recording information if it is in the first place not accurate. It is also important that systems are in place to enable the data to be kept up to date. An individual may change their name, address and many other things throughout their life.

Principle 5 – **"Personal data processed for any purpose or purposes shall not be kept for longer than is necessary for that purpose or those purposes".**

This has always been a grey area in radiology in general. How long should we keep x-rays for?

How long should we keep reports for? Previously these factors were determined by the availability of space for the storage of paper and x-ray film (with the associated problem of the long term tying up of silver resources).

These arguments will no longer hold because information that has been stored digitally can, if stored carefully, be kept for many years if not decades. However the x-rays on the disks may become irrelevant in less than a single decade. Do we then need to go back through our archives destroying data that is no longer relevant, and yet keep that which still is?

As more sectors of the health service become digitised these areas will be gradually addressed and guidelines drawn up. At the moment it is very much down to individual establishments to justify what they are doing.

Principle 6 – **"Personal data shall be processed in accordance with the rights of data subjects under this Act."**

This section highlights the rights of individuals under the Data Protection Act to prevent the processing of their data for several reasons. One example would be if it the processing of the data is likely to cause distress to the individual.

Principle 7 – **"Appropriate technical and organisational measures shall be taken against unauthorised or unlawful processing of personal data and against accidental loss or destruction of, or damage to, personal data."**

The potential always exist for information, especially digital to be accessed by unauthorised persons. Any establishment can only take so many steps to prevent this from happening, and they must be seen to do so. This can include firewalls, automated logout of workstations etc. However if a computer giant such as Microsoft is capable of being 'hacked' into then a hospital network must be considered to be equally vulnerable.

Systems to prevent the loss of data are also extremely important in a medical imaging department. If a high dose procedure such as a computed tomography (CT) scan of the thorax, abdomen and pelvis has been carried out and before it is archived or imaged it is deleted from the hard drive of the computer the entire procedure would have to be repeated with the associated increase in dose and stress to the patient.

Safeguards must be in place to ensure that this does not happen.

Principle 8 – **"Personal data shall not be transferred to a country or territory outside the European Economic Area, unless that country or territory ensures an adequate level of protection for the rights and freedoms of data subjects in relation to the processing of personal data."**

Whilst the ultimate aim is to ensure the secure and free transfer of data for legitimate purposes not all countries have standards that are equal to the United kingdoms so consideration of this must be made before transferring information to countries outside of the European Economic Area (EEA).

The Data Protection Act is not there to hinder modern imaging practices, but to ensure that the data is fairly used. It is important that any imaging department becomes familiar with it.

HEALTH AND SAFETY 1974

Source: http://www.hse.gov.uk/index.htm

This act has been amended several times to included new working practices. All employers should have a summary of the act displayed clearly and advising all staff who the Health and Safety Advisors are within the department.

The Health and safety regulations lay out the duty that an employer has to their employees and to the public who may come into a place or work. It also outlines the duty that the employees have to themselves and to each others.

A simple example might be that the employer is duty bound to provide a safe environment to work in and that the employees are duty bound to ensure that it remains safe. If a danger is noticed then something must be done about it immediately.

A key area in this process is risk assessment whereby the potential dangers are exposed and safety measure put in place to ensure that the risk is minimised or removed.

Any incident, including near misses must be reported to the Health and Safety representative in your department. This will normally include the filling in of a form, which the risk assessment team will forward to the Health and Safety Exec-utive if appropriate. Serious breeches of the act may result in prosecution of the managers under the act.

Health and Safety covers many areas including electricity and hazardous gases and so it is particularly applicable to hospital environments.

HEALTH AND SAFETY (DISPLAY SCREEN EQUIPMENT) REGULATIONS 1992

Source: http://www.hse.gov.uk/pubns/vduindex.htm
Source: http://www.hmso.gov.uk/si/si1992/Uksi_19922792_en_1.htm

One document that it is important to become particularly familiar with is the HS(DSE) regulations. If much of the radiographer of the future's work is going to be digital then much of our time will be spent looking at images on display screen equipment of one type or another.

The regulations outline what it is the responsibility of each employer to do in order to provide a safe working environment for those using display screen equipment. It should be remembered that DSE refers to all of the equipment used in displaying information and not just the monitor.

WORKING WITH DSE

Source: http://www.hse.gov.uk/pubns/indg36.pdf

This document outlines the basis of good practice in the use of display screen equipment (DSE). This document also refers to more than just DSE, incorporating all of the equipment used to aid in the display of information including the keyboard, mouse, table etc. This document outlines in understandable English the main considerations for the use of DSE. It is also an important document to have available for staff to read as it answers many of the most common questions asked by those using DSE.

HUMAN RIGHTS ACT 1988

Source: http://www.hmso.gov.uk/acts/acts1998/19980042.htm
Source: http://www.lcd.gov.uk/hract/hramenu.htm

This document is the UK application of the European Convention on Human Rights (ECHR).
http://www.echr.coe.int

This document outlines the basic rights of every human being as drawn up by the European Convention on Human Rights. The rights include such things as the right to life, the prohibition of torture, and prohibition of slavery amongst others. These basic human rights may only be over ruled if an act of parliament means that they must be.

The full extent of the impact (if any) of the Human Rights Act on medical imaging remains to be seen.

THE FREEDOM OF INFORMATION ACT 2000

Source: http://www.hmso.gov.uk/acts/acts2000/20000036.htm

This act deals with allowing the public access to information that is held by public authorities and is very similar in nature to the act that has existed in the United States for some years.

This act will come in to force in November 2002 and will allow a wide range of access to Government information. Its impact on other areas remains to be seen.

NHS SPECIFIC DOCUMENTS

ENSURING SECURITY AND CONFIDENTIALITY IN NHS ORGANISATIONS

Source: http://www.n-i.nhs.uk/dataprotect/action_plan/action.pdf

The Data Protection Act 1998 – An Action Plan

This is an NHSIA (see later) publication that seeks to clarify areas of the Data Protection for users within the NHS. It lists a plan of action enable establishments to examine their existing provision and where weaknesses may lay. It explores the eight principles with direct reference to the NHS and also list other documents that readers may wish to refer to for further information.

VDUser Friendly

This is a practical guide to the HS(DSE) and covers the problems that may be encountered during the installation and use of display screen equipment in a modern imaging department. Such practical guides are always helpful in understanding the more complex legal documents produced by the Government.

It is obtainable from the Society of Radiographers.

The NHS Plan

Source: www.nhs.uk/nhsplan
Quotes from: www.nhs.uk/nhsplan

The actual document is quite large so a summary document is also available. This is useful if used in conjunction with the full document to act as a reference for any points that require clarification or expansion.

It is important to at least become familiar with the basic principles, as they will have an effect on all working practices within the NHS of the future.

The main thrust is one of improving services to provide a "health service fit for the 21st century: a health service designed around the patient."

To this end there are several key changes to the way that the NHS must work.

- "More and better paid staff using new ways of working
- Reduced waiting times and high quality care centered on patients
- Improvements in local hospitals and surgeries."

These are very broad changes but they each have an impact on the delivery of health care in a modern imaging department and this is reflected in the following documents, which are specific to the delivery of information.

The document then highlights the problems in the current NHS and the ways in which these problems will be addressed and the level of investment that will accompany this reform. The need for full integration of services and the potential for role expansion in all areas is also explored as a further solution to problems and an improvement in the service delivered.

The need for wider do-operation with the private sector is outlined and this has implications for the sharing of digital information in the future and the security implication associated with it.

The reform is general in some respects and specific in others but the overall aim is to improve the delivery of health care at all levels and inherent within this will be the inevitable use of information management and technology to achieve these ends. Because of the importance of this area of NHS reform the NHS Information Authority was established.

The NHS Information Authority

Source: http://www.nhsia.nhs.uk/def/home.asp

The NHSIA was set up "as a special health authority, our remit is to enable the national infrastructure for an on-line NHS with electronic health records, an electronic library of knowledge, and the convenient services that people expect from a modern NHS" (www.nhsia.nhs.uk). The website is a wealth of information, documents and links to appropriate sites. For anyone involved in the development or use of information management and technology this site will be of great interest.

It contains links to many other documents, some of the key ones which will follow.

Information For Health

Source: http://www.nhsia.nhs.uk/def/pages/info4health/1.asp

This document sets out the Governments vision for delivering the best health care in the world to all of the population in the United Kingdom. To this end it recognizes the importance that information technology will play in this role.

It sets out several clear aims to enable this;

- The Electronic Health Record (EHR)
- 24 hour access to the EHR
- Seamless integration of data from different sources

- Online access of the public to information
- Effective access of staff to the information that they require

Adapted from: http://www.nhsia.nhs.uk/def/pages/info4health/1.asp

The document goes into great detail about how the IM&T strategy fits into the governments wider policy and the benefits of this to the nation. There are several key points to ensure an effective strategy.

- information will be person-based
- systems will be integrated
- management information will be derived from operational systems
- information will be secure and confidential
- information will be shared across the NHS.

Taken from: http://www.nhsia.nhs.uk/def/pages/info4health/1.asp

This pulls together all that has been said in previous chapters about the need for a single record (what in effect the EPR and EHR will be) that is fed information from many systems that are easily interfaced. Information can then be pulled from the system and shared as required providing it adheres to the Data Protection Act.

The document then outlines the needs of the various stakeholders within the NHS and the community and the need that may arise. Strategies for the implementation are then outlined.

At this point it is worth clarifying several key terms, the Electronic Patient Record (EPR) and the Electronic Health Record (EHR).

EPR & EHR

Initially the favoured term for the single source of patient information was the EHR, but this has changed now to provide two distinct records. They can be defined as follows.

EPR

The EPR will be a full record of all medical events that the patient has ever undergone, both in primary care (community) and secondary care (hospitals) institutions. It will effectively replace the patient's notes and will include the following elements;

- Written records of patient episodes which may be voice dictated and transcribed
- Images – histology, x-rays, photographs etc.

The system could also be expanded to store moving images

- Sound – the potential exists to store the spoken word, Doppler studies, heart sounds etc
- Waveforms – ECGs, EEGs etc.

The scope of the EPR will undoubtedly grow as the information available grows. A new benefit would be that incorporated into these would be community episodes to which the hospital staff would not have had immediate access. This would remove the need to rely on patients to tell the practitioner what treatment they are undergoing and what medication they are taking.

EHR

This will be a summary of patient episodes similar to the record kept by General Practitioners (GPs) at the moment. It would allow quick and easy access to pertinent points of a patient's records without having to filter through masses of information. This will enable GPs to carry out their work in the minimum amount of time.

Many GPs are already using electronic databases to record patient information and to print prescriptions, paving the way for a fully integrated system once the rest of the NHS catches them up.

But whilst these terms may come to be used there is also some notion of a more generic term, the electronic record, and it may be that the distinction between differing records will be lost.

The NHS Information Policy Unit

Source: http://www.doh.gov.uk/ipu/

This unit is responsible for the implementation of the NHS IT strategy and contains links to relevant information on information strategy along with guidance and updates as they are required.

Department of Health Documents

Source: www.doh.gov.uk/ipu/strategy/archive/index.htm

The Department of Health (DoH) also has several useful documents on Information Management and technology (IM&T) implementation and these can be found at the above web page that lists all of the related documents.

The NHS Information Management and Technology Strategy – Good Practice

Source: http://www.doh.gov.uk/ipu/strategy/archive/nhsboard.pdf

This document was produced in 1998 by the Enabling People Programme and sets out to explain the actual IM&T strategy with an aim to setting up standards of good practice that the whole NHS can use. It is actually aimed at board level employees but has much information that will be of interest to other individuals.

The government has recognised not only the need for a coherent approach to digital data within the NHS, but also its potential as a resource to reduce costs and increase effectiveness. To this end much work as gone into creating a strategy for the NHS to deal with the current levels of information and the future mass of information that will eventually be produced.

Consider for a moment the amount of data that your department would generate in one month. Then consider the amount of information that your hospital would generate, then all of your local hospitals, clinics, health centres and General Practitioner (GP) surgeries. Multiply this Nationwide and the volume of data that will be generated and transferred every day is likely to be huge, even by today's standards.

This document takes a series of simple questions that all hospitals should be asking themselves and then seeks to answer them with reference to the IM&T strategy. The standards it sets may seem obvious at times, such as the ideal that all patient information should only need to be inputted once. However this is rarely the case seen in the current NHS where patient data is often required to be inputted many times on different systems that are completely isolated with the network of the hospital.

This is a useful and practical document to peruse.

POISE

Source: http://www.pasa.doh.gov.uk/it_telecoms/poise/

The Purchasing and Supplies Agency of the NHS provides expertise in all areas of purchasing supplies and equipment for the health sector.

Their scope includes information technology equipment. POISE stands for Procurement Of Information Systems Effectively and is the UK standard for IT purchasing

PRINCE

Source: http://www.ogc.gov.uk/prince/about_intro.htm

PRINCE stands for PRojects IN a Controlled Environments and is the standard project management model used for information technology implementation in the UK. A new version known as PRINCE2 has now replaced the initial model.

Ionising Radiations Regulations 1999 (IRR99)

These came into force in January 2000 and they replace the Ionising Radiation Regulations of 1985 and cover the use of ionising radiations in al kinds of work places (hospitals, power stations etc) They are concerned with the responsibilities of both employers and employees. It is again an extensive document.

The employer must ensure a safe work place is provided for staff and the public, and the employees must maintain this safe environment and the people in it.

Important Points

- Dose limits are set for radiation workers and for members of the general public. The effective dose limit for radiation workers is 20 milliSieverts per year and for members of the public it is 1 milliSievert per year.
- Arrangements must be made for personal dosimetry for employees whose work is such that they may receive more than 3/10 of their dose limit.
- Any area in which radiation doses could exceed 3/10 of the relevant dose limit must be identified as a controlled area and entry into the controlled areas must be restricted.
- Within the work place a **radiation protection supervisor** (RPS) must be appointed from among the employees. The **RPS** is to take responsibility for ensuring, on a day-to-day basis, that the requirements of radiation protection are fulfilled. The RPS will ensure, for example, that radiation-warning lights are operating effectively, that dosimeters are

properly looked after and that new staff understand how to protect themselves when x-ray exposures are made. The RPS must have a good understanding of radiation protection and be sufficiently senior that the staff will respect their authority.
- This should not be confused with the **RPA** (radiation protecting advisor) who is a radiation expert − normally an experienced physicist.
- There must be written rules in each workplace to ensure that staff work within the law in relation to radiation protection. These rules are known as Local Rules. They must be brought to the attention of every employee and they must be displayed in a prominent place for all to see. They will include the names of the RPS and the RPA (if appointed), and they may identify rooms with in the practice where radiation protection must be applied and will outline particular precautions to taken when exposures are made in this room.
- The local rules apply the national legislation in the local situation. The national legislation states the requirements in very general terms, while the local rules are written specifically for the set of circumstances which exist in the work place. This should identify controlled areas.

The implications of IRR 99 is mainly on ensuring that the RPS and RPA are well informed on the impact of digital imaging on practice and thus local rules that were written for conventional systems may well need to be adapted to the new working environment.

Ionising Radiations (Medical Exposure) Regulations 2000 (IR(ME)R)

Source: www.doh.gov.uk/irmer.htm
Quotes from: www.doh.gov.uk/irmer.htm

Most radiography departments will be very familiar with the basic concepts within the IR(ME)R document. IR(ME)R replaces the Ionising regulations of 1998 (POPUMET) and came into force in May 2000. They protect the patient from unnecessary exposure to ionising radiations whilst undergoing medical examinations or treatment

- The new legislation defines the terms Referrers, Practitioners and Operators:
- "A referrer is a registered medical or dental practitioner, or other health professional who is entitled to refer individuals for medical exposure to a practitioner."
- "a practitioner is a registered medical or dental practitioner or health care professional who is entitled .... to take responsibility for an individual medical exposure."
- "An operator is any person who is entitled in accordance with the employers procedures to carry out any practical aspect associated with the procedure of a medical exposure."
- The Practitioner is responsible for justifying the medical exposure, but the operator is responsible for each and every practical aspect which they carry out and is required to apply the ALARP principle in respect to choosing the equipment and methods, paying particular attention to quality assurance and the assessment of patient doses.
- The legislation requires that employers ensure that every practitioner or operator is adequately trained and undertakes continued education and training after qualification.

RCR

The Royal College of Radiologists (RCR) is an invaluable source of information, much of which can be accesses online via www.rcr.ac.uk. Their main strength is that documents are produced that deal with subjects that are at the forefront of modern medical imaging and address the problems by drawing on the experiences of those that have already tackled the issues.

They are comprehensive and are updated as required. They are occasionally also joint publications with other bodies such as the Society of Radiographers (SOR) and the General Medical Council.

There are several documents that are related directly to the modern imaging department and links to them have been included that were correct at the time of writing.

Radiology Information Systems

Source: www.rcr.ac.uk/pubtop.asp?
PublicationID=142

This document deals with the importance of the Radiology Information System (RIS) in a radi-

ology department. If a fully integrated Picture Archiving and Communications Systems (PACS) to become possible the it must start with systems that allow the accurate storage of information and the retrieval and use of this information by other systems.

The initial aim of this document was to enable a department to develop a business case for a RIS that would fulfil the long term needs of an imaging department. One of the main thrusts is to ensure that any RIS that is introduced is able to support and enable other technologies such as PACS or tele-radiology which may at the moment seem a long way off but will be impossible with out a sound IT infrastructure.

The document takes a logical approach outlining all of the steps that are necessary to ensure a successful bid. Key areas are the advantages of having such a system and the benefits to the trust in potential costs and in reduced risk.

Practical applications are explored including the processes by which appointments etc are made and tracked through the system and the uses that this information must be able to be put to. Networking issues such as the exchange of information between a RIS and the Hospital Information System (HIS) are also explored, along with the impact that decisions might make.

From the combined experience of the authors of this book one of the key problems has been the issue of training the staff to use the system in not only a methodical way, but in a continuous fashion. This document also emphasise the importance of a training strategy in the successful implementation of a new RIS.

Where this document becomes particularly valuable is in its outline of the procedures that must be followed during the procurement procedure. If these rules are not closely followed then money will be wasted by having to return to areas that were not done properly the first time.

Other areas covered are how to cope with problems with the system.

Guide to Information Technology in Radiology, Tele-radiology and PACS. Second Edition

Source: http://www.rcr.ac.uk/pubtop.asp?
PublicationID=52

This document sets out to give guidance on the best way to enable tele-radiology and PACS.

It builds upon the advice offered in the first edition and it is recognised that this will not be the last edition as the field is constantly evolving.

Rather than saying exactly how things should be done it outlines what must happen for systems to be intra-operable. For example it does not explain exactly how various HL7 dialects should be translated into usable language by a PACS broker, rather it says that this is what must happen for the systems to talk and allow the exchange of information.

The document continues to outline the many issues that have been raised in this book such as the potential for DICOM to allow full integration, but its short comings at the moment. Issues such as bandwidth are discussed and the potential implications on an imaging service.

The document then spends much time discussing the intricacies of tele-radiology, its uses and potential problems. Similar attention is given to PACS along with a guide to building a business case including an analysis of benefits in terms of costs and reduced risks.

Newly included in this edition is the section on financing and the options that are available to those working within the NHS.

This is an essential document for those who are involved in any aspect of digital imaging, whether it be in procurement or in the actual implementation of a new system. Some interesting areas are then explored to which there are at the moment no clear answers. These include medico-legal issues and the potential for the internet as an enabling technology for tele-radiology.

Notes on Access to, Transfer and Storage of Patient Records created in Radiology Departments

Source: http://www.rcr.ac.uk/pubtop.asp?
PublicationID=53

This document explores the need for access to patients information in order that legal requirements under IR(ME)R, such as justification, can be achieved and through this reduce the number of unnecessary examinations and therefore dose that patients receive every year.

It notes that within the health service there is traditionally a lack of sharing in information and this needs to be addressed but only within the remit of the Data Protection Act 1998. Providing the eight principles are adhered to there should be nothing to prevent the appropriate disclosure of patient information to authorised sources, whether that data is digital or paper.

What makes up a record is then discussed which summarises many of the documents that have been produced by the government to give guidance. It is a practical application of the Caldicott report.

OTHER WEB SITES OF INTEREST

SOCIETY OF RADIOGRAPHERS

This site at the time of writing is under development and is expanding all of the time to provide a resource for radiographers and associated staff members. The site can be accessed by the public but full access requires membership of the Society of Radiographers. www.sor.org The monthly magazine of the Society of radiographers, Synergy, publishes articles on current topics including digital medical imaging

13: THE FUTURE OF DIGITAL IMAGING

Jason Oakley

INTRODUCTION

It is safe to say that the future of medical imaging is firmly digital, whether the changeover takes five or fifty years. The Government's policies for a better National Health Service (NHS) are driving this inexorably forwards. The potential benefits in having a fully integrated NHS electronic data system are many-fold and the technologies now exist to make the theory a reality.

Terminology will undoubtedly come and go as the NHS moves into a fully digital era. Already words such as 'systems' are being replaced by 'solutions', perhaps recognising that the installation of a system at the moment can constitute a complex interfacing problem. Whilst the terms electronic patient record (EPR) and electronic health record (EHR) are enshrined in Government policy the two terms have already caused some confusion and there is a move towards using the term 'electronic record' to define patient health data.

There is little doubt that computer systems will become more powerful, incorporate more RAM (random access memory) and be able to transfer data at far higher speeds. In the same way as personal computers seem to be constantly offering more for your money, medical imaging systems will be able to do the same as more systems come online and market acceptance of the technology increases. The competition for new business is already more intense that it was five years ago with many companies offering long term solutions to the handling and display of patient data.

The converse of this is the gradual phasing out of conventional film screen combinations. This may result in very few providers of conventional systems and a feeling of isolation for hospitals holding onto this technology because they are not part of the national Electronic Patient Record. There is little doubt that all health care providers will eventually be left with no option other than to manage patient information digitally.

This chapter will look at some of the issues that are currently considered important and others that are evolving in current digital medical imaging. However, from the time this chapter is completed, until the time you read it there will undoubtedly have been many advances in the world of computers and therefore in the world of modern radiography and radiology and this chapter will already be out of date.

ELECTRONIC PATIENT RECORD

Mention has already been made of the Electronic Patient Record (EPR) and its counter part the Electronic Health Record (EHR). The next ten years will see a complete move towards this, ensuring that hospitals with separate Hospital Information Systems (HIS), Radiology Information Systems (RIS) and imaging systems become fully integrated. The realisation that it is no longer adequate to have individual departmental systems has already changed the nature of the solutions that the manufacturers are supplying.

Many Picture Archiving and Communications Systems (PACS) are now being sold as 'Medical Image' solutions rather than Radiology department solutions. The manufacturers have been forced to look at the requirements of the management of health data for the benefit of the patient as a whole, rather than on an incident by incident basis. This has led to systems that are designed to incorporate patient notes, photographs, requests, histology, reports and of course radiology images.

The EPR has great potential for benefits to the NHS, such as being able to access all of the patient's information at any location in the United Kingdom (UK) but there are many issues that will have to be resolved. Some of these areas might be;

- Rights of access for levels of staff – decisions will have to be made on who should have access to what types of information and how the security of this data is assured. However, it is also important to ensure that in an emergency the data can be accessed quickly and freely.
- Rights of access for patients – this right is explicitly stated in the Data Protection Act (1998). With the increasing level of public access to the Internet the potential exist for all patients to be able to access their own records online, avoiding the time and admin-

istration issues associated with manually retrieving and showing patients their data.

- Rights of access for research – the potential using the EPR as a national database for research are enormous. When you consider that large cohorts are required to establish any link between exposure to diagnostic levels of radiation and disease the benefits are obvious. However, issues around the patient's consent for their information to be used in this way must also be considered
- Accuracy of data recorded – a major issue will be ensuring that data stored is accurate and up to date. This is a difficult problem to solve as there is now central record that could be used to update information nationally. A fully integrated system should at least mean that patient data only has to be inputted the first time they attend, at least reducing the points of failure to the minimum possible. The future may hold a national Identification card (something which many people are opposed to) and this may come with a requirement to inform the issuing body of any change in circumstances, name or address etc., and this type of database could be used to keep NHS information up to date.
- Unknown patients – How systems handle unknown patients and how this data can later be amalgamated with other data will be important.

These are only a few of the issues that will come to bear as a result of the Electronic Patient Record. As the record is implemented many more will undoubtedly appear.

POTENTIAL FOR HUMAN RIGHTS ISSUES

Much has been made of in the media of the inappropriate storage of human tissue within hospitals for research and other purposes. The ethical debate about the rights and wrongs of some of the practices will go on for some time, but one method of avoiding such situations is to utilise a digital archive. One of the main drives for digital imaging has been in histopathology where pattern recognition software can be used to identify what is 'not normal' for an experienced human viewer to look at.

Not only has this potentially removed the need to keep slides for long periods of time but it also makes recalling data simpler and far more reliable. A digital image that is stored appropriately should last beyond the life of any patient.

A side issue from this is that not everyone may be happy with their initial (or indeed final) diagnosis being made by a computer system. The NHS must decide what, if any, provision will be made for individuals that object to automatic screening. It may be that all that is needed is easy to understand evidence proving the increased sensitivity of computer systems over humans in the detection of the abnormal to remove the publics' fears.

It should also be possible for patients to dictate what they are happy for the data stored on them to be used for. The Data Protection Act (1998) states that patients must opt in, not opt out to any specific areas. A patient could be given a long list of tick boxes for them to agree to their data being used for everything or only certain things, in much the same way as organ donors can select only certain parts of their body to be used for donation.

If the management of patient information is not carried out with transparency and consideration the chances are that legal cases will be brought under either the Human Rights Bill or the Data Protection Act 1998.

PATTERN RECOGNITION

Much work is being done on the potential for computers to remove some of the errors that are introduced by humans interpreting medical images. Whilst no computer, at this time, can compete with a human on specificity (what a pathology actually is) they can compete in sensitivity (being able to tell that something is not 'normal'). Computers are also not affected by tiredness, hunger and cannot be distracted. This does not make them 100% reliable and the sensitivity and specificity of different systems will vary.

However, computers can be made use of to identify what is blatantly normal, and flag up only those that it is unsure of, thus reducing the volume of work that requires a human input. Because these images have been identified as potentially having an abnormality the human interpreter will be prepared to look at the images a little closer, which should reduce the error rate.

COMPRESSION

If the EPR is going to become a workable reality one of two things must happen; either file sizes must become smaller to allow realistic transfer times and display of patient information, or the method of data transfer must change. The potential for compression has been demonstrated (Image Manipulation and compression) but the resultant image degradation issues have not yet been evaluated.

Research is being carried out into many different types of compression algorithms and it is very possible that an effective method of compressing radiological images will be found that will vastly reduce the file size and allow much faster data transfer rates. The type of compression used may well be a wavelet type or may possibly come form the much-hyped potential for fractals to be used in the creation of images.

DATA TRANSFER

The other option to make the EPR realistic is to create a much faster "backbone" to the NHS intranet both on a national and local level. An improved network will allow faster data transfer for the storage and recall of data. The potentially huge amount of data that any such network would have to cope with makes the full EPR a huge undertaking.

Broadband connections are yet to take the UK by storm, but they will undoubtedly have a large impact on the home access Internet market, and may provide a solution to radiologists viewing images at home, but whether such a system is capable of supporting the massive data issues associated with a digital NHS remains to be seen.

COMPUTING POWER

The computer games industry drives the personal computer market forwards, pushing the need for increased memory, better graphics, improved visual displays, faster read/write times and faster processing power. The medical imaging community benefits from this by being able to access faster processors and increased amounts of memory.

Images are basically comprised of large amounts of data that take up a lot of memory. The more memory that is available, the more likely it is that the image we are looking at is displayed in the RAM that can be read far faster than the hard drive. If we wish to manipulate the image then we rely upon fast processor speeds to carry out the computations required to alter the image.

RAM is a relatively old technology and it is likely that in the near future new technology will become available that will make RAM even faster, larger and inexpensive.

It is worth noting that once it would have taken thirty minutes to physically go and get a set of old films that did not come with a patient. A wait of over twenty seconds is considered unacceptable on a computer system, with many wanting instant (less than 5 seconds) recall of old images. The demands we place upon a computer system are very different.

A question that can be easily justified is 'if it is not demonstrably better, then why are we changing?'

MEMORY

Computers come with ever increasing amounts of storage space in the form of hard drives. The technology that writes the tracks and sectors onto hard drives is reaching the point where no more information can be physically squeezed into the available space. This is driving the companies to search for a new solution to hard drive data storage. The next ten years will see a dramatic change in the way that computers store data, with an equally dramatic increase in the amount of data that they can store.

This change in technology may also result in an increase in the speed at which data can be written to and retrieved from the hard drive. This will enable far faster manipulation of large image files. An increased capability to store more data also means that longer periods of data can be stored directly online rather than in a portable medium such as magneto optical discs in a jukebox.

VISUAL DISPLAY EQUIPMENT

Only a few years ago the release of the affordable 15-inch monitor caused a degree of excitement amongst personal computer (PC) owners, but now 17 and 21-inch monitors are easily affordable.

Flat screen technology is progressing forward and market acceptance of this technology has meant that prices have come down bringing low quality flat screens into the home PC market. The technology is also improving meaning that manufacturing is cheaper, quality is better and the viewing angle of the screen is increased.

There is the potential for flat screen technology to continually improve with the screens becoming thinner and thinner and even being able to be shaped to a particular environment.

The potential also exists for the resurgence of the touch screen to replace the need for a keyboard. Fuji systems identification terminals (IDTs) already utilise this technology to improve the speed at which a film can be named and the appropriate algorithm applied to it.

WORKSTATION PLACEMENT

The affordability of high quality flat screen technologies means that visual display equipment can now be placed almost any where in the hospital environment. Flat screens are particularly useful in areas where the larger footprint of a traditional cathode ray tube (CRT) monitor would be obtrusive. Examples include the resuscitation room, operating theatres and nurse's stations.

FLAT PANEL DETECTORS

Under the chapter on equipment the difficulties in creating large flat panel detectors (FPDs) were discussed. Undoubtedly this technology will improve and larger plates will be constructed with less 'dead' space resulting in systems with a much higher detected quantum efficiency (DQE). The potential exists for entire x-ray table tops that double as detectors and intelligent systems that know which part of the table has been exposed.

Digital radiography systems will become fully portable and may move away form the current systems that require the replacement of the x-ray tube and other associated pieces of equipment.

The potential for rapid acquisition using flat panel detectors is already being utilised in fluoroscopic units. Units will be available with the image intensifier being replaced by a FPD making the unit smaller and easier to move. These will be incorporated into departmental fluoroscopic systems and will reduce the dose to the patient whilst increasing image quality. Such systems can be more easily incorporated into computed tomography (CT) scanning machines to allow dual imaging during complex procedures.

WIRELESS SYSTEMS

The imaging suite of the future will not require cables to connect the FPDs to the computers. Instead the image will be sent in a digital stream, using infra-red technology, directly to the computer. This technology could make theatre work even easier with no cables on the floor of the operating theatre. Major users of x-rays, such as ITU, could have their own terminal to which the plate is pointed to be read. The image then almost instantaneously appears on the monitor whilst the radiographer is still on the unit. Simultaneously a radiologist and a specialist can be viewing the image in another building.

Wireless technology also means that images could be sent to a specialist anywhere in the world providing that the specialist is carrying appropriate receiving equipment. The possibilities are limitless.

TELERADIOLOGY

As handheld devices become of better quality and telecommunications networks improve there can be no doubt that this technology can be used to greatly enhance the service that the diagnostic imaging department provides to the patient. By utilising technologies that will allow the remote viewing of images faster specialist advice can be sought at any time of the day or night.

This technology will also allow these specialists a degree of freedom whilst on call, not requiring them to remain near a fixed computer terminal and phone line. Teleradiology will undoubtedly play a huge part in the future of radiography and radiology.

VIRUSES

There is little doubt that at some point a virus will infect a hospital system. It may be a very minor incursion with minimal loss of data or it could be catastrophic. Whichever it might be the future will see a continuing battle between those creating viruses and those attempting to protect systems from them.

HEALTH ONLINE

NHS Direct has been of some success but one of the main problems has been getting the target groups within society to use the telephone as a means of obtaining health information. In the same way online facilities for patients can only help those who are online and know where to find the information.

The Government has an agenda to ensure that all households have access to the Internet by 2005, and one way of achieving this has been to introduce digital television that comes with a simple browsing facility built in. This removes the unfamiliar computer system and replaces it with something that the majority of the country is all too familiar with, a television.

The potential, though, is for a much larger part of the population to be reached via the Internet with health information. There is also some scope for communication with patients via e-mail and for them to check appointment times, seek advice on their procedure and check any worries they may have online. At the moment the security problems with e-mails prevent this from being a secure medium of communication.

As resources become ever more stretched computers will be relied upon to reduce the burden to the clinicians by allowing patients to self diagnose or by filtering appropriate patients to other professionals.

HEALTH INFORMATICS

Health Informatics (HI) is going to become an important part of the health service agenda. HI has many definitions, but in the modern NHS it can be considered to be the methods of managing data using computers. The potential uses and benefits that may be gleaned from the effective management of this information are huge, and the Government recognises this fact.

Two bodies, the NHS Information Authority (NHSIA) and the Information Policy Unit at the Department of Health (DoH IPU) have been established to ensure that the EPR happens and that it happens in a way that ensures maximum benefits can be made from the available information.

NEW TECHNIQUES

Whilst much of the new technology sought to merely replace the existing film/screen combinations with a filmless alternative there will certainly be new techniques that are made possible by the new technology. An example of this might be dual energy x-ray techniques where a low kV and high kV chest x-ray are acquired in rapid succession using a flat panel detector. These two images can be subtracted from each other to produce a image that shows the bony anatomy and another that appears to have had the rib-cage removed and thus clearly shows all of the lungs.

This is but one example of a new technique that has been enabled by digital radiography.

CONCLUSION

Whatever the future may hold for radiography and radiology it will certainly be an exciting place to be, despite the many problems that are associated with the installation, interfacing and acceptance of these new technologies. It will be a period where the importance of Continuing Professional Development (CPD) will be paramount if radiographers, radiologists and other health care professionals are to keep abreast of the latest developments.

This book has hopefully explored the area

from beginning to end and those who started with no knowledge will feel that they have a grasp of the methods and technologies that are shaping modern medical imaging. Those that already had a certain amount of knowledge will know more and also know where to deepen their knowledge.

The importance of the imaging department in the diagnosis and treatment of patients has never been underestimated, but now the potential exists for its role to expand until it will become a fully integrated part of all working environments in any hospital. In ten years the health care professionals will look back in wonder that it took thirty minutes to return a portable x-ray to the ward, an hour to get old films sent up to a ward and that the possibility existed that films might actually be lost.

GLOSSARY

ACR	American College of Radiologists
ADSL	Asymmetrical Digital Subscriber Line – method of sending receiving large amounts of data (downstream) and transmitting less data (upstream) utilising POTS
AET	Application Entity Title in DICOM
ALU	Arithmetic Logic Unit – controls advanced mathematical functions to free up CPU time
Analogue	Being made up of a continuously changing waveform
Application	Software that performs a specific task, such as Microsoft word
ASCII	American standard code for information interchange
ATM	Asynchronous Transfer Mode
Bandwidth	Digital – the amount of data that is transmitted in bits per second (bps)
	Analogue – expressed in cycles per second (Hz)
Binary	Numbers in the base of 2 i.e. 2^n
BIOS	Basic Input/Output system – contained within the computers ROM and allows the computer to turn on.
Bit	Smallest component of binary data. Term derived from binary digit.
Boot	The program stored in the systems ROM that starts the computer up. Supposedly from the term 'to pull yourself up by your bootstraps'.
bps	Bits per second (occasionally bytes per second – Bps)
bus	Connection between two parts of the computer
Byte	Eight bits of information form one byte of information. All subsequent multiples are worked out from bytes e.g. kilobyte. Will have a most significant and least significant nibble.
CCD	Charge Coupled Device
CD-ROM	Compact Disc Read Only Memory – inexpensive data distribution media.
CD-R	Compact Disc Recordable – inexpensive data recording media which utilises a dye, burnt by a laser, to record digital information. Not erasable or re-recordable
CD-RW	Compact Disc ReWritable – data recoding media that utilises crystals whose appearance can be changed from reflective to dull by heating with a laser. Erasable and rewritable.
CPU	Central Processing Unit – controls all of the functions of the computer
CR	Computed radiography – normally referring to phosphor storage plate technologies
CRT	Cathode ray tube – traditional technology for emitting electrons. Utilised in standard monitors and televisions.
CT	Computed Tomography
DDR	Direct Digital Radiography – normally refers to direct acquisition technologies
DICOM	Digital Image Communication in Medicine

Digital	Being made up of binary information.
DIMSE	DICOM service Message Element
Direct Access Storage	Storage media where the read device can go straight to the data without having to spool through other data
DMWL	DICOM Modality Work List
DoH	Department of Health
DQE	Detected Quantum Efficiency – a measure of the quality of an image
DR	Digital Radiography – normally referring to indirect acquisition technologies
Electro-mechanical	A device that combines electronics and mechanics to carry out a function
FDD	Floppy Disk Drive
FDDI	Fibre Distributed Data Interface – a type of token ring network running on fibre optic cables
Firewall	Network equipment to insulate one network from another one, for example insulating the hospital's network from the rest of the internet.
HL7	Health Level 7 - a standard for interfacing Health related information systems together.
Hexadecimal	Numbers in base 16. Used to deal with very large numbers on a computer
Hard copy	A physical representation of either ext or images. Laser film is an example of this, as is the printed word.
Hard drive	Magnetic permanent rewritable memory of the computer
HIS	Hospital Information System
Histogram	Graph showing the number of pixels per grey level
HTML	Hyper-Text Mark up Language – the computer language used to create and view document on the www.
IP	Internet Protocol – as in IP Address
ISDN	Integrated Service Digital Network
LAN	Local Area Network – normally a small network connecting PCs within a small area.
LAS	Large Average Signal – the average pixel value of an image
LASER	Light Amplification of Stimulated Emission of Radiation
LCD	Liquid Crystal Display
Lossless	Normally refers to compression techniques that do not lose any image quality
Lossy	Normally refers to compression techniques that irreversibly lose image quality
LR	Limiting resolution
MAC address	A number allocated to every piece of network equipment. It is fixed and no two MAC addresses are ever the same.
Magneto	Utilising a magnetic field

Magneto-optical	Utilising a magnetic field and light to carry out a function
Manipulation	Method of changing the appearance of an image using filters or mathematics
Matrix	Number of pixels in the x and y direction
MRI	Magnetic resonance imaging
MTF	Modulation Transfer Function − a measure of the original frequency amplitude compared to the output
NEB	Noise Equivalent Bandwidth
NEMA	National Electrical Manufacturers Association
NHS	National Health Service
NHSIA	National Health Service Information Authority
NM	Nuclear medicine
NPS	Noise Power Spectrum (Weiner Spectrum)
Nyquist Frequency	Rate of sampling required to represent the highest frequency with the image (2f)
Optical	Utilising light
OS	Operating System − e.g. Windows NT, 98, Unix etc.
OSI	Open Standards Interconnect - a structured way of layering the different tasks network equipment must do in order to communicate.
PACS	Picture Archiving and Communication System
PACS Broker	Interface engine for HL7 and DICOM common data such as name, patient number etc
Pixel	Picture element, normally described by the function f(x,y)
PMI	Patient Master Index
POST	Power On Self Test − performed by every computer during a cold start
POTS	Plain Old Telephone Service − existing copper wire telephone network
QA	Quality Assurance
RAM	Random Access Memory − fast but volatile temporary memory
RCR	Royal college of Radiologists
RIS	Radiology Information System
RPM	Revolutions Per Minute
SCP	Service Class Provider in DICOM
SCU	Service Class User in DICOM
SMPTE	Society of Motion Picture and Television Engineers
SNR	Signal to Noise Ratio − ratio of background random data to actual signal
Soft copy	This is the image displayed on the computer which has no physical presence (unlike film, which is hard copy)
SOP	Service Object Pair in DICOM

SoR	Society of Radiographers
TCP	Transmission Control Protocol
TFT	Thin film transistor
Token Ring	A type of network arranged in a ring and using tokens to indicate if the network can be written to.
UPS	Un-interruptible power supply – used to allow a controlled shut down during a power failure
URL	Universal (Uniform) Resource Locator – a unique address for every web site and web page.
US	Ultrasound
UTP	Unshielded Twisted Pair - a type of network cable that connects your computer to the network.
Virtual Memory	Hard drive memory that is used to carry out functions if the RAM is already full
Voxel	A pixel that also has depth, such as is acquired during a CT scan
WAN	Wide Area Network – normally covering a large area and involving two or more LANs. The world wide web for example.
WORM	Write Once Read Many – many storage media (see CD-R) are permanent and once the data has been written and the full capacity of the media used the data cannot be erased of written over. Data can be read again and again.
www	World Wide Web – The largest WAN, incorporating the vast number of connected servers all using html.

MCQ SECTION

INTRODUCTION

This chapter has been included in an attempt to fulfil the need for health care professionals to not only to seek to improve themselves, but also to record their learning as evidence of their continuing education. It is recommended that you complete this section after reading and assimilating each of the chapters. Record your results as part of your continuing medical or professional education and revisit areas that you are weak in. This section can be revisited again and again until you are happy that your knowledge meets your needs.

The answers to each section are found at the end in a format that should allow quick marking.

MCQ 1 – CHAPTER TWO – THE BASICS

Q		T	F	DK
1	The term decimal refers to working in base 10	☐	☐	☐
2	It is easy for computers to work using decimal code.	☐	☐	☐
3	There are 8 bits to a byte	☐	☐	☐
4	1 megabyte is exactly 1,000,000 bytes	☐	☐	☐
5	A bit depth of 2^8 would give 512 different variables	☐	☐	☐
6	The characters on the keyboard conform to the ASCII code	☐	☐	☐
7	Hexadecimal is used because binary code can be too short	☐	☐	☐
8	An analogue wave form is made of discrete values	☐	☐	☐
9	A digital signal is more reproducible than an analogue signal	☐	☐	☐
10	The sampling rate of a signal should be twice the highest frequency within the object being imaged	☐	☐	☐
11	A digital image is made up of a continuous waveform	☐	☐	☐
12	A colour image will have double the number of bits than its black and white counterpart	☐	☐	☐
13	A voxel is a pixel that had depth (z) as well as x,y dimensions	☐	☐	☐
14	An image file is comprised of two distinct data components	☐	☐	☐
15	A look up table is referred to by the user to check the images grey scale	☐	☐	☐
16	In an unwritten magnetic tape the magnetic domains are randomly orientated	☐	☐	☐
17	Recording onto digital tape and analogue tape are the same thing	☐	☐	☐
18	Analogue bandwidth is determined by the Hz of the system	☐	☐	☐
19	High digital bandwidth is determined by the speed of the connection	☐	☐	☐
20	Computed radiography can reduce doses by a factor of ten when compared to traditional film/screen combinations	☐	☐	☐

MCQ 2 – CHAPTER THREE – EQUIPMENT A

Q		T	F	DK
1	CT, MRI, US and Nuclear Medicine are not digital imaging modalities	☐	☐	☐
2	An IBM compatible PC and a MAC PC are the same thing	☐	☐	☐
3	A device that protects a computer from power loss or power surge is known as a UPS	☐	☐	☐
4	The mother board of a computer is a bracket for the attachment of circuitry	☐	☐	☐
5	The CPU of a computer is the control unit for all activity in the computer	☐	☐	☐
6	The ALU is the Additional Latitude Unit	☐	☐	☐
7	RAM is a form of permanent memory	☐	☐	☐
8	The BIOS contains all the information to start the computer	☐	☐	☐
9	A BUS is a moving component within a computer	☐	☐	☐
10	PCI stands for peripheral components interconnect	☐	☐	☐
11	Secondary memory refers to the volatile memory of a computer	☐	☐	☐
12	Controller cards tell the CPU what to do	☐	☐	☐
13	A buffer stores data going to a peripheral device to allow the CPU to return to other functions	☐	☐	☐
14	A sound card is basically a digital to analogue converter and vice versa	☐	☐	☐
15	A graphics card is a device for drawing on	☐	☐	☐
16	A network card controls the exchange of information between the computer and the network it is connected to	☐	☐	☐
17	A modem is solely an analogue device	☐	☐	☐
18	A traditional serial port is the fastest type of connection	☐	☐	☐
19	Parallel ports are two ports next to each other	☐	☐	☐
20	USB stands for Universal Serial Bus	☐	☐	☐

MCQ 3 – CHAPTER THREE – EQUIPMENT B

Q		T	F	DK
1	A keyboard is an electro-mechanical input device	☐	☐	☐
2	A mouse is a purely mechanical device	☐	☐	☐
3	Barcodes cannot be used to store text information	☐	☐	☐
4	The operating system controls the running of the computer	☐	☐	☐
5	An application is a form of operating system	☐	☐	☐
6	GUI stands for Graphical User Input	☐	☐	☐

Q		T	F	DK
7	File size has no impact on the time the file will take to transfer	☐	☐	☐
8	There is a big difference in the time different storage media take to read and write data	☐	☐	☐
9	Data written in one format can always be read by other systems	☐	☐	☐
10	Cost effectiveness is all about purchasing the cheapest solution	☐	☐	☐
11	A 3.5 inch floppy disk is ideal for storing medical images	☐	☐	☐
12	Floppy disks are a magnetic storage system	☐	☐	☐
13	Floppy disks utilise direct access storage	☐	☐	☐
14	The computer has to search through the whole of the floppy disk to find the file requested	☐	☐	☐
15	If you open a computer up it is possible to see the platters of the hard drive	☐	☐	☐
16	A hard drive is a direct access storage media	☐	☐	☐
17	Magnetic tape is a direct access storage media	☐	☐	☐
18	A CD-ROM can be written to many times	☐	☐	☐
19	A laser is utilised to record data on a recordable CD	☐	☐	☐
20	CDs are an indirect access storage media	☐	☐	☐

MCQ 4 – CHAPTER THREE – EQUIPMENT C

Q		T	F	DK
1	A DVD can only store double the data that a CD can	☐	☐	☐
2	DVDs are a direct access storage media	☐	☐	☐
3	A magneto optical system utilises a laser to heat up magnetic domains	☐	☐	☐
4	Magneto optical systems are less robust than CD and DVD technology	☐	☐	☐
5	A juke box is a device for playing music in scanning suites	☐	☐	☐
6	All monitors are of the same quality	☐	☐	☐
7	Cathode ray tubes utilise a stream of electrons to stimulate a phosphor screen	☐	☐	☐
8	Colour phosphor screens are brighter and of a higher resolution than monochrome phosphors	☐	☐	☐
9	A shadow mask and aperture grill fulfil the same function	☐	☐	☐
10	Gas plasma displays are limited to monochrome displays	☐	☐	☐
11	Liquid crystals change shape when an electric current is passed through them	☐	☐	☐
12	A passive display is brighter than an active display	☐	☐	☐
13	Dot pitch is the size of a single phosphor grain	☐	☐	☐
14	The traditional monitor size given is its diagonal measurement	☐	☐	☐

Q		T	F	DK
15	This diagonal measurement is still suitable for diagnostic imaging	☐	☐	☐
16	The number of pixels that a monitor can display has no effect on image quality	☐	☐	☐
17	Any display device can display an image at full resolution by magnifying it	☐	☐	☐
18	Luminance is higher in monochrome monitors	☐	☐	☐
19	A low refresh rate will cause the monitor to flicker	☐	☐	☐
20	CRT monitors are lighter than their flat screen counterparts	☐	☐	☐

MCQ 5 – CHAPTER THREE - EQUIPMENT D

Q		T	F	DK
1	CR stands for computed radiography	☐	☐	☐
2	Static electricity can effect photo-stimulable phosphor	☐	☐	☐
3	Phosphor storage plates only come in one speed	☐	☐	☐
4	Resolution is given in lp/mm in two directions	☐	☐	☐
5	A laser emits an incoherent beam of light	☐	☐	☐
6	A latent image is effectively stored in the phosphor plate	☐	☐	☐
7	CR systems have some inherent unsharpness	☐	☐	☐
8	CR cassettes do not require erasure	☐	☐	☐
9	The term DR refers to indirect digital radiography	☐	☐	☐
10	DR cassettes are more robust than CR cassettes	☐	☐	☐
11	DR systems are theoretically sharper than CR systems	☐	☐	☐
12	DR systems are theoretically sharper than DDR systems	☐	☐	☐
13	CR systems are less expensive than DR and DDR systems	☐	☐	☐
14	CCD stands for Charge Coupled Device	☐	☐	☐
15	TFT stands for Terrifically Fine Transmitters	☐	☐	☐
16	DR and DDR are faster than CR	☐	☐	☐
17	All printers are of equal quality	☐	☐	☐
18	Hard copy technologies are no longer needed	☐	☐	☐
19	Dry processing technologies are environmentally friendly	☐	☐	☐
20	Image quality is higher on hardcopy than on a monitor	☐	☐	☐

MCQ 6 – CHAPTER FOUR – INTERFACE STANDARDS

Q		T	F	DK
1	A standard is the same as a file format	☐	☐	☐
2	The first solely digital device was the MRI scanner	☐	☐	☐
3	DICOM stands for Digital Imaging and Communications in Medicine	☐	☐	☐
4	Systems from different manufacturers can be connected easily	☐	☐	☐
5	Future proofing is ensuring that files can be read for the life time of the media	☐	☐	☐
6	The header of a data file contains the image information	☐	☐	☐
7	Images are normally stored in decimal format	☐	☐	☐
8	Lossy compression does not result in any loss of image quality	☐	☐	☐
9	DICOM is an evolving standard that changes all of the time	☐	☐	☐
10	New modalities cannot be added to the DICOM standard	☐	☐	☐
11	DICOM is a set of instructions to allow communication	☐	☐	☐
12	DICOM utilises fields to ensure that each system knows where each piece of information will be	☐	☐	☐
13	HL7 deal with images and not text	☐	☐	☐
14	ISO OSI stand for International Standards Organisation Operating System Interconnect	☐	☐	☐
15	The aim of HL7 is similar to DICOM, that is to ensure effective communication	☐	☐	☐
16	HL7 does not split information into fields	☐	☐	☐
17	A device for enabling communication is called an interface engine	☐	☐	☐
18	HL7 and DICOM are global standards	☐	☐	☐
19	IHE stands for Integrating Health Enterprise	☐	☐	☐
20	A systems that says that it is HL7 or DICOM compliant will definitely be able to communicate with another system	☐	☐	☐

MCQ 7 – CHAPTER FIVE – NETWORKS

Q		T	F	DK
1	Interfacing is what makes PACS come alive	☐	☐	☐
2	A network is the physical method of connection between systems	☐	☐	☐
3	A network cannot be made of anything other than copper wires	☐	☐	☐
4	A network uses a low voltage to represent a 1 and no voltage to represent 0	☐	☐	☐
5	A network card is different from a network interface card	☐	☐	☐
6	The speed of a network is measure in Mb/s	☐	☐	☐

Q		T	F	DK
7	UTP stands for Universal twisted pair	☐	☐	☐
8	CR images take up little network time	☐	☐	☐
9	An IP address is individual to every piece of equipment in an institution	☐	☐	☐
10	A collision occurs when two systems send information at the same time	☐	☐	☐
11	A hub connects individual networks	☐	☐	☐
12	Routers control access of information to the correct parts of the networks	☐	☐	☐
13	A switch is an intelligent hub	☐	☐	☐
14	An interface engine automatically inputs data	☐	☐	☐
15	A PACS broker is a device for DICOM to HL7 conversion and vice versa	☐	☐	☐
16	DMWL stands for DICOM modality work list	☐	☐	☐
17	Interfacing increases the number of input errors	☐	☐	☐
18	PACS does not need to communicate with HIS	☐	☐	☐
19	Interfacing is easy to achieve	☐	☐	☐
20	Networks will frequently need upgrading	☐	☐	☐

MCQ 8 – CHAPTER SIX – RIS

Q		T	F	DK
1	RIS is the same as PACS	☐	☐	☐
2	It is important to have a good knowledge of RIS	☐	☐	☐
3	A proprietary RIS is guaranteed to use HL7	☐	☐	☐
4	Interfacing an HL7 RIS to another HL7 system can still be difficult	☐	☐	☐
5	Paper systems are more reliable than digital systems	☐	☐	☐
6	Digital information has far more uses	☐	☐	☐
7	Research is one of the main areas to benefit from the digital storage of data	☐	☐	☐
8	A RIS can only operate on a proprietary terminal	☐	☐	☐
9	Future proofing is about ensuring that the equipment lasts as long as possible	☐	☐	☐
10	PMI stands for Patient Message Interface	☐	☐	☐
11	An interface engine translates the data from one system into a format that another can deal with	☐	☐	☐
12	Data entry is the biggest single contributing factor to system errors	☐	☐	☐
13	It is easy to find a patient on the system if their data has been inputted incorrectly	☐	☐	☐
14	Order communications deals with queuing patients in the department	☐	☐	☐
15	A log on password (electronic signature) is less important than a written signature	☐	☐	☐

Q		T	F	DK
16	Cross site appointment booking is not possible with RIS	☐	☐	☐
17	All staff should have access to all areas of the RIS	☐	☐	☐
18	It is vital that all events in any patient episode can be traced to an individual	☐	☐	☐
19	RIS terminals are not affected by the Health and Safety Act (Visual Display Equipment)	☐	☐	☐
20	A RIS will last indefinitely and never need upgrading	☐	☐	☐

MCQ 9 – CHAPTER SEVEN – PACS

Q		T	F	DK
1	One of the main benefit of PACS is the simultaneous viewing of an image in multiple locations	☐	☐	☐
2	PACS can only deal with radiological images	☐	☐	☐
3	PACS can only operate on a single site	☐	☐	☐
4	Storage is not a major consideration for traditional film based radiology	☐	☐	☐
5	The local set up will determine the design of the PACS	☐	☐	☐
6	A UPS is essential to prevent power surges	☐	☐	☐
7	PACS is solely radiology's concern and should not involve the wider hospital	☐	☐	☐
8	CR or DR must be able to run independently of the PACS	☐	☐	☐
9	PACS is readily accepted by all staff	☐	☐	☐
10	Key areas to involve in consultation are A&E, ITU and Orthopaedics	☐	☐	☐
11	PACS requires a network of its own	☐	☐	☐
12	Existing equipment such as CT scanners cannot be linked into the PACS	☐	☐	☐
13	Contingency plans for unplanned down time are essential	☐	☐	☐
14	IP addresses are Identifying Pathway addresses	☐	☐	☐
15	Additional equipment can be added at a later date providing it can be made to interface	☐	☐	☐
16	DICOM is the only type of information that the PACS can handle	☐	☐	☐
17	A PACS Broker buys second hand PACS from hospitals	☐	☐	☐
18	A RAID is a relatively cheap way of storing large amounts of data	☐	☐	☐
19	PACS implementation may require a transitional period from traditional to digital	☐	☐	☐
20	Perceptions of downtime with PACS are different from perceptions of downtime with traditional equipment	☐	☐	☐

MCQ 10 – CHAPTER EIGHT – IMAGE PROCESSING

Q		T	F	DK
1	An image can be represented by the function f(x,y)	☐	☐	☐
2	An analogue image is made up of discrete values	☐	☐	☐
3	PIXEL stands for picture element	☐	☐	☐
4	The size of a matrix is not determined by binary code	☐	☐	☐
5	The sampling rate does not affect image quality	☐	☐	☐
6	The Nyquist frequency is double the lowest frequency in an image	☐	☐	☐
7	A grey level histogram depicts the quantity of each grey scale within an image	☐	☐	☐
8	Any image can be made from combining different waveforms	☐	☐	☐
9	Image manipulations can be carried out only in the spatial domain and not the frequency domain	☐	☐	☐
10	Point operations are used to combine images	☐	☐	☐
11	Local operations are used to combine images	☐	☐	☐
12	Fourier transform is a global operation	☐	☐	☐
13	A high pass filter removes high frequencies	☐	☐	☐
14	Image segmentation divides a picture in half	☐	☐	☐
15	Lossy compression loses no image quality	☐	☐	☐
16	All compression ratios give the same quality image	☐	☐	☐
17	Redundant data is information that is repeated such as background data	☐	☐	☐
18	Huffman encoding allocates the shortest binary numbers to the most common grey scales	☐	☐	☐
19	JPEG is the only form of compression available	☐	☐	☐
20	Compression cannot cause artefacts	☐	☐	☐

MCQ 11 – CHAPTER NINE – IMAGE QUALITY

Q		T	F	DK
1	Image quality is easy to measure and to assess	☐	☐	☐
2	Spatial resolution is the smallest distance between two objects that can be measured	☐	☐	☐
3	Matrix size and pixel size must both be known to measure image quality	☐	☐	☐
4	Voxel size has no affect on image quality	☐	☐	☐
5	All parts of the imaging chain will have the same effect on image quality	☐	☐	☐
6	High noise and low contrast make a good image	☐	☐	☐

Q		T	F	DK
7	Low noise and high contrast make a good image	☐	☐	☐
8	Grey scale response ensures that all display devices present the image in the same way	☐	☐	☐
9	Dynamic range defines how fast an imaging device acquires an image	☐	☐	☐
10	Noise can be completely removed from any system	☐	☐	☐
11	MTF stands for Modulation Transfer Function	☐	☐	☐
12	MTF is usually stated at 20%	☐	☐	☐
13	Aliasing is caused by over sampling an image	☐	☐	☐
14	DQE is a measure of the overall quality of a system	☐	☐	☐
15	You cannot give a CR plate too little exposure	☐	☐	☐
16	QA does not need to be carried out on the imaging plates	☐	☐	☐
17	Printers are prone to artefacts which need to be recognised	☐	☐	☐
18	Quality assurance tests are easy to carry out	☐	☐	☐
19	The implementation of PACS will have a large impact on the amount of QA required	☐	☐	☐
20	QA is not a valuable use of time	☐	☐	☐

MCQ 12 – CHAPTER TEN – COMMONLY USED PARAMETERS

Q		T	F	DK
1	Brightness and contrast should be adjusted using the monitor settings	☐	☐	☐
2	Utmost care must be taken when altering any patient information	☐	☐	☐
3	It is no longer important to ensure correct markers are on the film at time of exposure	☐	☐	☐
4	All images will require manipulation of some kind	☐	☐	☐
5	Automatic shuttering can subjectively improve an images quality	☐	☐	☐
6	Correct image orientation is of little importance	☐	☐	☐
7	Histograms can be used to analyse the properties of an image	☐	☐	☐
8	Soft tissue filters increase the contrast in an image	☐	☐	☐
9	Trabecular bone is less detailed on a soft tissue filter	☐	☐	☐
10	Softening an image removes the edges within it	☐	☐	☐
11	Softened images are more pleasing to the human eye	☐	☐	☐
12	Edge detection increases the subjective appearance of bone	☐	☐	☐
13	Harsh edges are more pleasing to the human eye	☐	☐	☐
14	Response curves can be altered by the user	☐	☐	☐

Q		T	F	DK
15	Response curves do not predict what the final image will look like	☐	☐	☐
16	The response curve for an inverted image is the opposite of the normal response curve	☐	☐	☐
17	An inverted image contains more information than the original	☐	☐	☐
18	There is a time advantage to using preset parameters	☐	☐	☐
19	Measurements cannot be reliably made on the computer	☐	☐	☐
20	There is no place for individual image manipulation	☐	☐	☐

MCQ 13 – GENERAL QUESTIONS A

Q		T	F	DK
1	Websites remain active indefinitely	☐	☐	☐
2	The internet is a secure method of communication	☐	☐	☐
3	The Data Protection Act (1998) applies to medical images	☐	☐	☐
4	Patients must opt in to any options, not opt out	☐	☐	☐
5	Informed consent is no longer an issue	☐	☐	☐
6	Digital images should be kept forever	☐	☐	☐
7	DSE stands for Department of Social Economics	☐	☐	☐
8	Health and safety is very important in modern imaging departments	☐	☐	☐
9	Guidance notes are more important than the original documents	☐	☐	☐
10	The web base documents are the definitive version	☐	☐	☐
11	Ensuring that you are up to date with Government Policy has never been so important	☐	☐	☐
12	The European Computer Driving Licence is not relevant to the NHS	☐	☐	☐
13	The Government has no long term strategy for information technology in the NHS	☐	☐	☐
14	IR(ME)R is even more important in the digital imaging field	☐	☐	☐
15	Radiographers should be part of any procurement team	☐	☐	☐
16	The web is of little use to the modern practitioner as a source of information	☐	☐	☐
17	Storage of data is major issue for imaging departments	☐	☐	☐
18	User tolerance decreases as technology becomes faster	☐	☐	☐
19	There is no need for health care professionals to be trained in how equipment works	☐	☐	☐
20	Continuing professional development has never been so important	☐	☐	☐

MCQ 14 – GENERAL QUESTIONS B

Q		T	F	DK
1	Security is not an issue for a radiology department	☐	☐	☐
2	All users should have equal access	☐	☐	☐
3	Patients have the right to see all information kept on them	☐	☐	☐
4	Radiographers are all computer literate	☐	☐	☐
5	Training on new systems should be continuing	☐	☐	☐
6	Workload is normally decreased with the incept of a PACS system	☐	☐	☐
7	Ambient viewing conditions do not affect the apparent image quality on a monitor	☐	☐	☐
8	Repetitive Strain Injury does not occur from using a computer	☐	☐	☐
9	A CR system can produce a good image from a vastly over-exposed cassette	☐	☐	☐
10	DR systems allow a rapid turn over of patients	☐	☐	☐
11	CR systems require the complete replacement of all x-ray equipment	☐	☐	☐
12	CR removes the need to consider exposure factors	☐	☐	☐
13	It is essential that all users within the hospital are involved in consultation processes	☐	☐	☐
14	The main advantage of CR systems is dose reduction	☐	☐	☐
15	Quality Assurance for digital systems is well established	☐	☐	☐
16	Compression of images can be done without worry	☐	☐	☐
17	Computers will change beyond recognition in the next ten years	☐	☐	☐
18	Tele-medicine is unlikely to have a major impact in the UK	☐	☐	☐
19	Interaction and communication with radiology departments will alter significantly	☐	☐	☐
20	The future is bright	☐	☐	☐

ANSWERS

MCQ 1 – Chapter two – The Basics

Q	T	F
1	✓	
2		✓
3	✓	
4		✓
5		✓
6	✓	
7		✓
8		✓
9	✓	
10	✓	
11		✓
12		✓
13	✓	
14	✓	
15		✓
16	✓	
17		✓
18	✓	
19	✓	
20		✓

MCQ 2 – Chapter three – Equipment a

Q	T	F
1		✓
2		✓
3	✓	
4		✓
5	✓	
6		✓

Q	T	F
7		✓
8	✓	
9		✓
10	✓	
11		✓
12		✓
13	✓	
14	✓	
15		✓
16	✓	
17		✓
18		✓
19		✓
20	✓	

MCQ 3 – Chapter three – Equipment b

Q	T	F
1	✓	
2		✓
3		✓
4	✓	
5		✓
6		✓
7		✓
8	✓	
9		✓
10		✓
11		✓
12	✓	
13	✓	
14		✓
15		✓
16	✓	

Q	T	F
17	☐	✓
18	☐	✓
19	✓	☐
20	☐	✓

MCQ 4 – Chapter three – Equipment c

Q	T	F
1	☐	✓
2	✓	☐
3	✓	☐
4	☐	✓
5	☐	✓
6	☐	✓
7	✓	☐
8	☐	✓
9	✓	☐
10	✓	☐
11	✓	☐
12	☐	✓
13	☐	✓
14	✓	☐
15	☐	✓
16	☐	✓
17	✓	☐
18	✓	☐
19	✓	☐
20	☐	✓

MCQ 5 – Chapter three – Equipment d

Q	T	F
1	✓	☐
2	✓	☐

Q	T	F
3	☐	✓
4	✓	☐
5	☐	✓
6	✓	☐
7	✓	☐
8	☐	✓
9	✓	☐
10	☐	✓
11	✓	☐
12	☐	✓
13	✓	☐
14	✓	☐
15	☐	✓
16	✓	☐
17	☐	✓
18	☐	✓
19	✓	☐
20	☐	✓

MCQ 6 – Chapter four – Interface Standards

Q	T	F
1	☐	✓
2	☐	✓
3	✓	☐
4	☐	✓
5	✓	☐
6	☐	✓
7	☐	✓
8	☐	✓
9	✓	☐
10	☐	✓
11	✓	☐

Q	T	F
12	✓	
13		✓
14	✓	
15	✓	
16		✓
17	✓	
18		✓
19	✓	
20		✓

MCQ 7 – Chapter five – Networks

Q	T	F
1	✓	
2	✓	
3		✓
4	✓	
5		✓
6	✓	
7		✓
8		✓
9	✓	
10	✓	
11		✓
12	✓	
13	✓	
14		✓
15	✓	
16	✓	
17		✓
18		✓
19		✓
20	✓	

MCQ 8 – Chapter six – RIS

Q	T	F
1		✓
2	✓	
3		✓
4	✓	
5		✓
6	✓	
7	✓	
8		✓
9		✓
10		✓
11	✓	
12	✓	
13		✓
14		✓
15		✓
16		✓
17		✓
18	✓	
19		✓
20		✓

MCQ 9 – Chapter seven – PACS

Q	T	F
1	✓	
2		✓
3		✓
4		✓
5	✓	
6	✓	
7		✓
8	✓	
9		✓
10	✓	

11	☐	✓
12	☐	✓
13	✓	☐
14	☐	✓
15	✓	☐
16	☐	✓
17	☐	✓
18	✓	☐
19	✓	☐
20	✓	☐

MCQ 10 – Chapter eight – Image Processing

Q	T	F
1	✓	☐
2	☐	✓
3	✓	☐
4	☐	✓
5	☐	✓
6	☐	✓
7	✓	☐
8	✓	☐
9	☐	✓
10	☐	✓
11	☐	✓
12	✓	☐
13	☐	✓
14	☐	✓
15	☐	✓
16	☐	✓
17	✓	☐
18	✓	☐
19	☐	✓
20	☐	✓

MCQ 11 – Chapter nine – Image Quality

Q	T	F
1	☐	✓
2	✓	☐
3	✓	☐
4	☐	✓
5	☐	✓
6	☐	✓
7	✓	☐
8	✓	☐
9	☐	✓
10	☐	✓
11	✓	☐
12	☐	✓
13	☐	✓
14	✓	☐
15	☐	✓
16	☐	✓
17	✓	☐
18	☐	✓
19	✓	☐
20	☐	✓

MCQ 12 – Chapter ten – Commonly used parameters

Q	T	F
1	☐	✓
2	✓	☐
3	☐	✓
4	☐	✓
5	✓	☐
6	☐	✓
7	✓	☐
8	☐	✓

Q	T	F
9	✓	
10	✓	
11	✓	
12	✓	
13		✓
14	✓	
15		✓
16	✓	
17		✓
18	✓	
19		✓
20		✓

Q	T	F
15	✓	
16		✓
17	✓	
18	✓	
19		✓
20	✓	

MCQ 14 – General Questions B

Q	T	F
1		✓
2		✓
3	✓	
4		✓
5	✓	
6		✓
7		✓
8		✓
9	✓	
10	✓	
11		✓
12		✓
13	✓	
14		✓
15		✓
16		✓
17	✓	
18		✓
19	✓	
20	✓	

MCQ 13 – General Questions A

Q	T	F
1		✓
2		✓
3	✓	
4	✓	
5		✓
6		✓
7		✓
8	✓	
9		✓
10		✓
11	✓	
12		✓
13		✓
14	✓	

Results

MCQ 1 – Chapter Two – The Basics   ....

MCQ 2 – Chapter Three – Equipment A   ....

MCQ 3 – Chapter Three – Equipment B   ....

MCQ 4 – Chapter Three – Equipment C   ....

MCQ 5 – Chapter Three – Equipment D   ....

MCQ 6 – Chapter Four – Interface standards   ....

MCQ 7 – Chapter Five – Networks   ....

MCQ 8 – Chapter Six – RIS   ....

MCQ 9 – Chapter Seven – PACS   ....

MCQ 10 – Chapter Eight – Image Processing   ....

MCQ 11– Chapter Nine – Image Quality   ....

MCQ 12 – Chapter Ten – Commonly used parameters   ....

MCQ 13 – General Questions A   ....

MCQ 12 – General Question B   ....

INDEX

Note: References to figures are indicated by 'f' when they fall on a page not covered by the text reference.